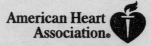

American Heart
Association®

Fighting Heart Disease and Stroke

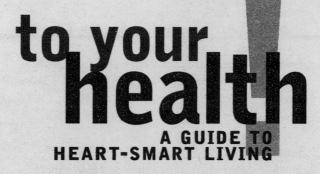

to your
health!

A GUIDE TO
HEART-SMART LIVING

Also by the American Heart Association

The New American Heart Association Cookbook, 25th Anniversary Edition

American Heart Association Low-Salt Cookbook, Second Edition

American Heart Association Low-Fat, Low-Cholesterol Cookbook, Second Edition

American Heart Association Quick & Easy Cookbook

American Heart Association Meals in Minutes Cookbook

American Heart Association Around the World Cookbook

American Heart Association Low-Fat & Luscious Desserts

American Heart Association Kids' Cookbook

American Heart Association Guide to Heart Attack Treatment, Recovery, and Prevention

American Heart Association Family Guide to Stroke Treatment, Recovery, and Prevention

Living Well, Staying Well: The Ultimate Guide to Help Prevent Heart Disease and Cancer (with the American Cancer Society)

American Heart Association 6 Weeks to Get Out the Fat

American Heart Association Fitting In Fitness

American Heart Association 365 Ways to Get Out the Fat

American Heart Association Brand-Name Fat and Cholesterol Counter, Second Edition

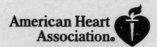

American Heart
Association®

Fighting Heart Disease and Stroke

to your
health!

A GUIDE TO
HEART-SMART LIVING

American Heart Association
Clarkson Potter/Publishers

New York

Your contribution to the American Heart Association supports research that helps make publications like this possible. For more information, call 1-800-AHA-USA1 (1-800-242-8721) or contact us online at www.americanheart.org.

Published by Clarkson Potter/Publishers, New York. Member of the Crown Publishing Group, a division of Random House, Inc.

www.randomhouse.com

CLARKSON N. POTTER is a trademark and Potter and colophon are registered trademarks of Random House, Inc.

Printed in the United States of America

Design by Jan Derevjanik

Library of Congress Cataloging-in-Publication Data
American Heart Association.
American Heart Association: to your health: a guide to heart-smart living / American Heart Association.
p.   cm.
1. Health.   2. Weight loss.   3. Smoking.   4. Heart—Diseases—Prevention.   I. Title.
RA776 .A425 2001
613—dc21   2001034354

ISBN: 0-609-80702-1

10 9 8 7 6 5 4 3

First Edition

American Heart Association Science Consultant: Terry Bazzarre, Ph.D.
American Heart Association Consumer Publications Director:
   Jane Anneken Ruehl
American Heart Association Science Editor: Ann Melugin Williams
American Heart Association Senior Editor: Janice Roth Moss
American Heart Association Editor: Jacqueline Fornerod Haigney
American Heart Association Editorial Coordinator:
   Roberta Westcott Sullivan
American Heart Association Volunteer Advisers: Lora Burke, Ph.D., Ruth Ann Carpenter, M.S., Nancy Houston-Miller, R.N., Rebecca Mullis, Ph.D.

CONTENTS

INTRODUCTION

EVERY YEAR IT'S ALWAYS THE SAME. YOU MAKE STUNNING RESOLUTIONS TO lose weight, get more exercise, or quit smoking—sometimes all three. January turns into June, though, and you find yourself struggling into last year's swimsuit, which now fits like a sausage casing. Maybe you still find yourself exhausted from exertion—and all you're doing is taking out the garbage! Even worse, you're inescapably tied to your next cigarette—even when you hate the idea of smoking.

"What's wrong with me?" you ask. "I've seen other people trim down and look great . . . I've seen them take up an active sport or hobby and get fit . . . I've seen them kick the smoking habit for good and feel tremendous relief. Why can't *I* make a fresh start?"

The simple truth is that these other people were *ready*. They realized what they really wanted and went after it. You can do it too, and this book will tell you how. It's all a matter of knowing what it takes to genuinely *want* to change your life. When you really want change, making it happen is actually quite simple. Why? Because you're working *for*—rather than *against*—your own true happiness.

At the American Heart Association, we believe in change—changing behavior to stay healthy. Every day, people around the world discover the secret to changing their life, and their health, for the better. Now you can do it too. In this book, we've included all the basics: everything you'll need to take stock, discover what you really want, uncover your personal barriers, and start a simple, step-by-step plan that will result in the healthier life you've always wanted. We've also included motivational tips for your overall health: how and why to take your medications and the benefits of getting regular medical checkups.

If an active, healthy, smoke-free life is what you've always wanted, we're ready to help you get there—one smart step at a time. *Here's to your health!*

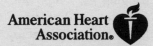

American Heart Association®

Fighting Heart Disease and Stroke

to your health!

A GUIDE TO HEART-SMART LIVING

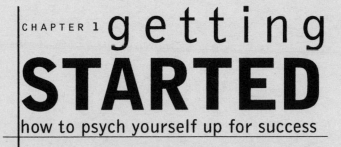

CHAPTER 1 getting
STARTED
how to psych yourself up for success

"WE HAVE MET THE ENEMY,
AND HE IS US."

— POGO

ALTHOUGH IT MAY BE TEMPTING TO SKIP THIS CHAPTER, *DON'T DO IT*. You may be thinking, "Get on with it. I want to lose twenty pounds. Just tell me how, and I'll do it." Trouble is, that's *not* how you lose 20 pounds—and keep it off. That's *not* how you quit smoking—and stay a nonsmoker. Instead, that quick-fix attitude is the recipe for failure, so stick with us here. This chapter is about the *inner* you, the single greatest key to changing your life.

Attitude Adjustment

The opening quote from Pogo reflects the heart of the problem. When it comes to getting what you want in life, you are your own worst enemy. Sure, others can help sabotage your efforts, and they often will, but your own double-mindedness is what allows that to happen. You are the captain of your fate—thinking anything else is sheer delusion.

Ralph is a perfect example. He was overweight as a child and obese as an adult. A therapist pointed out how as a child Ralph became a compulsive eater, and he embraced that idea at once. He grabbed at this truth, seeing it as *the* reason he was hopelessly fat. He decided that his overweight condition was fundamentally unchangeable—that it was his fate.

"I was miserable. Whenever I tried to lose weight, I failed. I thought nothing I could do would help, and sure enough, it never did," Ralph said. "I can see now that, in a sense, my attitude made me comfortable. The idea that I was powerless to change took the responsibility off my shoulders."

Ralph's comfort level hit the skids when he bumped into a buddy from his old weight-loss group. The man had lost 64 pounds and toned up well at the gym. Ralph almost didn't recognize him.

"This guy had a background similar to mine," said Ralph. "I realized that if he could do it, I could too. And, frankly, I wanted that kind of body. So all of a sudden, I realized there's no such thing as unchangeable fate—not when it comes to body weight. I had already proved that I could *increase* my body weight by any amount. Now I was determined to prove that I could *decrease* it by any amount."

Ralph asked for his buddy's eating plan and joined a gym. It took almost a year of trial and error, but Ralph went from 240 pounds to 175. After he lost the weight, he never went back to his old eating habits. He stuck with his weight-loss eating plan but added enough calories to keep his new weight stable.

"I have this pair of pants from my old days at 240," said Ralph. "I keep them because they remind me of something really important: I—and I alone—am responsible for my size. I determine my own fate."

How Badly Do You Want This?

Sure, you want to quit smoking. Who wouldn't? Your friends barely put up with it. Strangers are disgusted by it. You have about a million burn marks on your clothes, car, and furniture. And just buying the cigarettes costs enough to finance a yearly trip to Tahiti. Even so, you don't quit. Secretly, you may feel that you're just weak and you have no willpower. A lack of willpower is not the problem. You have all the willpower in the world. We believe that you're not really *ready* to quit. Deep down, you *just don't want to do it*.

That's okay. However, if you've picked up this book, we suspect that you're at least thinking about making a change. The book may nudge you in the right direction by giving you new information that will influence you to change. Or it may furnish you with tips on small changes that can ease you into a new course of action.

After reading the pertinent chapter, if you don't really want to lose weight, get more exercise, or quit smoking, put this book down until you do. If you're not ready, you'll be spinning your wheels and getting nowhere.

The first order of business is to determine whether you *really want* to make a change. Fortunately, that's easy. Everyone moves naturally through five stages on the way to lifestyle changes.

To find out which stage you're in, take the following Stages of Change Test. It will show where you are.

stages of change test

Circle the number that applies to your status.

a. SMOKING

1. I am currently smoking, and I do not intend to quit in the next six months.

2. I am currently smoking, but I intend to quit in the next six months.

3. I am currently smoking, but I intend to quit in the next month.

4. I have not smoked for the past six months.

5. I quit smoking more than six months ago.

6. I have never smoked, and I am confident that I never will.

b. HEART-HEALTHY DIET *

1. I am not eating a heart-healthy diet, and I do not intend to adopt one in the next six months.

2. I am not eating a heart-healthy diet, but I intend to adopt one in the next six months.

3. I am not eating a heart-healthy diet, but I intend to adopt one in the next month.

4. I have been eating a heart-healthy diet for less than six months.

5. I have been eating a heart-healthy diet for more than six months.

6. I have been eating a heart-healthy diet for more than six months, and I am confident that I will continue this diet no matter what roadblocks come up.

c. PHYSICAL ACTIVITY **

1. I am not physically active, and I do not intend to become active in the next six months.

2. I am not physically active, but I intend to become more active in the next six months.

3. I am not physically active, but I intend to become more active in the next month.

4. I have been physically active for less than the past six months.

5. I have been physically active for more than the past six months.

6. I have been physically active for more than six months and I am confident that I can continue no matter what roadblocks come up.

Find the number you circled for each of the behaviors listed above.

a. Smoking   _____
b. Heart-Healthy Diet   _____
c. Physical Activity   _____

Using the following key, rank your stage of change for each of the areas described above.

* *A heart-healthy diet contains less than 10 percent of daily calories from saturated fat, less than 300 milligrams of cholesterol per day, and less than 6 grams of salt per day.*

** *Physically active people are defined here as people who do at least 30 minutes of activities such as brisk walking, jogging, biking, or swimming at least three days each week.*

stages of change

1. YOU'RE NOT EVEN THINKING ABOUT IT. You haven't considered taking any steps to change the way you're eating, start exercising, or quit smoking.

2. YOU'RE THINKING ABOUT IT. You're considering making some changes but still haven't done anything.

3. YOU'RE GETTING READY. You're intent on changing, and you've even started to make a few inroads. You may have asked your friends about eating plans or called a quit-smoking clinic for information. You may have purchased some walking shoes, but they're still sitting in your closet.

4. YOU TAKE ACTION. You've begun the new eating plan. You've enrolled in the quit-smoking program. You've laced up your shoes and started walking.

5. YOU EMBRACE MAINTENANCE. You've been incorporating these lifestyle changes into your life successfully for a while, and you're starting to feel comfortable with them.

6. YOU'VE BEEN LIVING A HEALTHFUL LIFESTYLE FOR AT LEAST SIX MONTHS. Now you can't imagine your life any other way.

You cannot will yourself to move from one stage to another. But if you're stuck at one stage and wish you could move up a notch, there are some things you can try.

Perhaps you don't really understand the risks of your current behavior or the benefits of changing it, so you're stuck in Stage 2. If so, seek information about those risks and benefits. This book will help (see specifically the section you need to work on, and check out "Information Highway" on page 227).

You might be trapped at Stage 3 because you lack the confidence that you can make the needed changes. This book can help you gain that confidence by breaking the changes down into small steps that you can try. Once you try a step and succeed, you can move on to the next step. If you still need an extra boost, try working with a personal trainer, a registered dietitian, or a stop-smoking counselor. These professionals may be able to help give you the confidence you need.

Another aid to change is social support. Get a walking buddy or join a class. Sometimes seeing a friend take action helps you realize that you can do it too.

What's Your HQ (Health Quotient)?

It's difficult to get where you're going if you don't know where you are. That's why we created the following health-risk awareness questionnaire. It's designed to give you an idea of your overall health, especially your risk of heart attack or stroke. You may think you need to lose weight, quit smoking, or get more exercise. Maybe, though, other factors are really what you need to pay attention to most. Talk with your doctor if you feel you are at high risk of having a heart attack or stroke.

health risk
awareness test

The following factors may increase your risk of heart attack or stroke. Check all the items that apply to you. If you check two or more items on this test, you need to contact your health-care provider for a *complete health assessment*.

When it comes to heart attack or stroke:

Your AGE may increase your risk if:

___You're a man over 45 years old.

___You're a woman over 55 years old *OR* you have passed menopause or had your ovaries removed and you are not taking estrogen.

Your MEDICAL HISTORY may increase your risk if:

___You have coronary heart disease *OR* you've had a heart attack.

___You've been told that you have carotid artery disease *or* you've had a stroke or a transient ischemic attack (TIA) *or* you have a disease of the leg arteries.

Your FAMILY HISTORY may increase your risk if:

___Your father, brother, mother, or sister has had a heart attack.

___You have a close blood relative who has had a stroke.

Cigarette and tobacco SMOKE increases your risk if:

___You smoke *or* you live or work with people who smoke every day.

Your TOTAL BLOOD CHOLESTEROL and HIGH-DENSITY LIPOPROTEIN (HDL) CHOLESTEROL levels may increase your risk if:

___Your total cholesterol level is 240 milligrams per deciliter (mg/dl) or higher.

___Your HDL ("good") cholesterol level is lower than 40 mg/dl.

___You don't know your total cholesterol or HDL levels.

Your BLOOD PRESSURE may increase your risk if:

__Your blood pressure is 140/90 millimeters of mercury (mm Hg) or higher OR you've been told your blood pressure is too high.

__You don't know what your blood pressure is.

PHYSICAL INACTIVITY may increase your risk if:

__You don't get a total of 30 minutes of physical activity at least three to four days each week.

Excess BODY WEIGHT may increase your risk if:

__You're 20 pounds or more overweight for your height and build.

DIABETES increases your risk if:

__You have diabetes or you have a fasting blood sugar of 126 mg/dl or higher OR you need medicine to control your blood sugar.

health risk awareness test results

IF YOU CHECKED AGE, MEDICAL HISTORY, OR FAMILY HISTORY

See your family physician for an overall checkup if you haven't had one in the past year, especially if you're 65 or older; that's the age group in which over 70 percent of heart attacks occur. People who have a heart attack before 65 often have a strong family history of heart disease or stroke. If you have had a heart attack, you're at greater risk of having another.

IF YOU CHECKED SMOKING

Smoking is the single greatest preventable cause of death in the United States. The sooner you quit smoking, the sooner you'll lower your risk. For more information on how to quit, see our smoking chapter, page 161.

IF YOU CHECKED BLOOD CHOLESTEROL

Many studies show that for a person with blood cholesterol of 240 mg/dl or higher, the risk of heart attack is substantially greater than for a person whose cholesterol is 200 mg/dl. Have your cholesterol levels checked by a health-care provider. If your total cholesterol is 240 mg/dl or higher, or if your HDL cholesterol is lower than 40 mg/dl, discuss with your doctor how diet, exercise, and weight loss can improve your situation. Some people may also need medications that can help lower total cholesterol levels.

IF YOU CHECKED BLOOD PRESSURE

One in four adults in the United States has high blood pressure. That translates to about 50 million people. High blood pressure is often called the silent killer because it usually has no symptoms yet can result in heart attack or stroke. In fact, high blood pressure is the single most important risk factor for stroke. If you have high blood pressure, you may need to change your diet, lose weight, become more active, and also take medicine to get your blood pressure back to normal. If you drink alcohol, you may need to cut back to no more than one drink a day.

IF YOU CHECKED PHYSICAL INACTIVITY

One of the best things you can do for your health is get off your couch. Choose activities you enjoy and be sure you get a total of 30 minutes of physical activity three or more days a week to get started. Physical activity will help reduce your risk of heart disease, stroke, and diabetes. It also helps lower blood pressure and blood cholesterol. Read all about the benefits in our physical activity chapter, page 115.

IF YOU CHECKED BODY WEIGHT

Obesity is a risk factor for five of the ten leading causes of death in the United States: heart disease, stroke, high blood pressure, diabetes, and some types of cancer. Losing 10 to 20 pounds can help lower high blood pressure and total blood cholesterol and help control diabetes in some people. (*Caution: This book is not intended for people who need to lose 100 pounds or more, nor is it for those with binge-and-purge disorders. These two groups need medical supervision.*)

IF YOU CHECKED DIABETES

Several other risk factors for heart attack and stroke interact in diabetes. Obesity and physical inactivity are also risk factors for diabetes. Your blood pressure should be lower than 130/85 mm Hg. To control diabetes, you may need to change your eating habits, lose weight, increase your physical activity level, and even take drugs. It's critically important to have regular checkups.

latrice's story:
FOLLOW DOCTOR'S ORDERS

"I found out by accident that I have diabetes," said Latrice, a 22-year-old college student. "I went with a friend to the pharmacy. They were offering free screenings for diabetes, so we thought we'd do it just to see what happened."

To Latrice's amazement, the technician told her to make an appointment with her doctor for further screening. "I was totally caught off guard," Latrice said. "I was due for a checkup anyway, so I made an appointment right away."

Latrice met with her doctor the following week and was put on a special diet. "Fortunately, I had been thinking of making some lifestyle changes anyway. I had gained about fifteen pounds and wanted to get the weight off before I gained any more," Latrice said. "I decided to be optimistic about changing my life. I knew I had two choices: I could make the changes my doctor recommended or go on insulin and maybe have severe medical problems in the future. For me, it was no contest— I chose to follow my doctor's orders."

Latrice made the changes in her diet and then gradually added exercise. She has lost

20 pounds and manages her diabetes through diet, exercise, weight control, and medication. Because she made the decision to change her way of life, she has had no problem following her special diet and keeping the weight off.

Let's Get **Physical**: Regular Checkups

If nothing else, a regular checkup will give you several important numbers—your blood pressure; your total blood cholesterol, LDL cholesterol, and HDL cholesterol levels; and your blood glucose (sugar) level. Because your numbers can change at any time, your doctor should check your blood pressure during every office visit. If your blood cholesterol is at the desirable level, you should have it checked every 5 years until about age 45. If you're older than 45, get it checked every 2 years. If your blood cholesterol is high, check it at least *every year,* or more often if your doctor is monitoring your treatment.

THE HIGHS AND LOWS OF BLOOD PRESSURE

Everybody has—and needs—blood pressure. Without it, blood can't circulate through the body, giving vital organs the oxygen and food they need.

Under normal conditions, your heart beats about 60 to 80 times a minute. Your blood pressure rises with each heartbeat and falls when your heart relaxes between beats. Like the air pressure in your tires, your blood pressure can change from minute to minute. The pressure in your tires depends on the temperature and whether you've been driving. Your blood pressure changes with posture, exercise, sleeping, or even the level of your arm when the blood pressure is measured (the cuff should be level with your heart). A blood pressure measurement has two numbers:

1. The higher (systolic) number represents the pressure when the heart contracts.

2. The lower (diastolic) number represents the pressure when the heart relaxes between beats.

The systolic pressure is always stated first, and the diastolic pressure second. For example, a blood pressure of 122/76 is stated "122 over 76." The systolic is 122; the diastolic is 76.

When you're sitting at rest, your blood pressure should be lower than 130/85 millimeters of mercury (mm Hg) to be considered normal. A blood pressure reading equal to or higher than 140/90 is considered high. Therefore, if your systolic pressure is 130 to 139 or if your diastolic pressure is 85 to 89, it should be watched carefully.

High blood pressure is more common among people over thirty-five years old. It is more prevalent in African Americans, middle-aged and elderly people, obese people, heavy drinkers, and women who are taking birth control pills. Although high blood pressure can run in families, some people with a strong family history never have it. People who have diabetes, gout, or kidney disease are more likely to have high blood pressure than those who don't.

RECOMMENDED BLOOD PRESSURE LEVELS

CATEGORY	BLOOD PRESSURE SYSTOLIC	(mm Hg)	DIASTOLIC
Ideal* • Recheck in 2 years	Less than 120	*and*	Less than 80
Normal • Recheck in 2 years	Less than 130	*and*	Less than 85
High normal • Recheck in 1 year	130 to 139	*or*	85 to 89
High stage 1 • Confirm within 2 months	140 to 159	*or*	90 to 99
High stage 2 • Evaluate within 1 month	160 to 179	*or*	100 to 109
High stage 3 • Evaluate immediately	180 or higher	*or*	110 or higher

* *Your doctor should evaluate unusually low readings. If you have diabetes, heart failure, or certain kidney problems, your doctor will want your blood pressure to be in the ideal or normal range.*

Have your blood pressure taken and compare it to the recommended blood pressure levels on the previous page. Work with your health-care provider to control your blood pressure if it's too high or too low.

CHOLESTEROL: ARE YOUR NUMBERS UP?

Everyone's blood contains cholesterol. This waxy, fatlike substance is necessary for your body's cells. You need a small amount of cholesterol to make certain hormones, as well as cell membranes and other tissues. The trouble comes when you have too much cholesterol in your blood, because that's a major risk for heart disease. In turn, the accumulation of plaque inside the arteries in the heart can lead to blocked vessels and a heart attack.

Your body gets cholesterol in two ways. Your liver makes some of it—in fact, enough to meet your body's needs. The rest comes from animal products that you eat, such as meat, poultry, fish, eggs, butter, cheese, and whole milk. Foods from plants don't contain cholesterol.

Remember that saturated fat raises your blood cholesterol and LDL cholesterol (the "bad" cholesterol) more than anything else in the food you eat.

LDL AND HDL CHOLESTEROL

Cholesterol can't dissolve in the blood, so it must be transported to and from the cells by special carriers called lipoproteins. Two major kinds are low-density lipoprotein, or LDL (the "bad" cholesterol carrier), and high-density lipoprotein, or HDL (the "good" cholesterol carrier).

LDL cholesterol is called bad because LDL carries cholesterol *to* your arteries. Too much of it can clog the arteries to your heart and increase your risk of heart attack. HDL cholesterol is called good because it helps protect you. You can think of HDL as a garbage truck: It carries cholesterol away from your arteries and back to the liver for disposal, so a high level of HDL cholesterol in your blood reduces your risk of heart attack.

YOUR CHOLESTEROL LEVELS

If you have a high total cholesterol, you'll want to know three numbers: your total cholesterol level, your LDL cholesterol level, and your HDL cholesterol level. Have your doctor measure these levels regularly to make sure they're in the safe range. If they're not, work with your doctor, nurse, or dietitian to reduce your total cholesterol and LDL cholesterol levels and raise your HDL cholesterol levels. Check your blood cholesterol levels here:

- Desirable: less than 200 mg/dl

- Borderline high risk: 200 to 239 mg/dl

- High risk: 240 mg/dl or higher

If your cholesterol level is in the desirable range (less than 200 mg/dl)

Your risk of heart attack is relatively low unless you have other risk factors. Even so, it's still smart to eat foods low in saturated fat and cholesterol and get plenty of physical activity. Have your cholesterol levels measured every 5 years or, if you're a man older than 45 or a woman older than 55, every 2 years. Almost half the adults in the United States have total cholesterol levels lower than 200 mg/dl.

If your cholesterol is in the borderline high-risk range (200 to 239 mg/dl)

About a third of American adults have a borderline high-risk level. Have your cholesterol, LDL cholesterol, and HDL cholesterol rechecked in one to two years if your HDL cholesterol is 40 mg/dl or higher and you don't have other risk factors for heart disease.

Meanwhile, eat fewer foods high in saturated fat or cholesterol to reduce your cholesterol level to less than 200. Also see "Your LDL Cholesterol Level," page 24.

If your cholesterol level is in the high-risk range (240 mg/dl or higher)

Your total cholesterol level is definitely high risk. The higher your cholesterol, the greater your risk of heart attack and, indirectly, of stroke. Your doctor will want to test your blood for LDL and HDL cholesterol levels and discuss treatment with you. You're not alone. About 20 percent of the U.S. population have high-risk blood cholesterol.

YOUR LDL CHOLESTEROL LEVEL

The lower your LDL cholesterol, the lower your risk of heart attack and stroke. Your LDL cholesterol is an even better gauge of risk than your total blood cholesterol. When you have your LDL cholesterol checked, it will fall into one of these categories:

- Desirable: less than 130 mg/dl

- Borderline high risk: 130 to 159 mg/dl

- High risk: 160 mg/dl or higher

If your LDL cholesterol is too high, your doctor will likely recommend an eating plan low in saturated fat and cholesterol, regular exercise, and weight loss if you're overweight. If these don't lower your LDL cholesterol, your doctor can also prescribe medications to help reduce it.

YOUR HDL CHOLESTEROL LEVEL

In the average man, HDL cholesterol levels range from 40 to 50 mg/dl. In the average woman, they range from 50 to 60 mg/dl. An HDL cholesterol level that's less than 40 mg/dl puts you at high risk for heart disease. Smoking, being overweight, and having a sedentary lifestyle can all contribute to low

HDL cholesterol. If you have low HDL cholesterol, you can help raise it by:

- Not smoking

- Maintaining a healthy weight

- Being physically active for 30 to 60 minutes a day 3 or 4 days a week

- Avoiding anabolic steroids and male sex hormones (testosterone), which lower HDL cholesterol levels. Estrogen and other female sex hormones raise HDL cholesterol levels.

---

megan's story:
BE PROACTIVE IN YOUR MEDICAL CARE

"High blood pressure runs in my family, so it was no surprise when they put me on medication," said Megan, a 25-year-old writer. "I did, however, find it surprising that because of my age, even though the numbers showed that I had high blood pressure, doctors were reluctant to say I had it."

Because of her family history, Megan knew the dangers of high blood pressure. "I decided to take charge of my condition. I bought a monitor so I could check my blood pressure at home," Megan said. "I had been told that my blood pressure was high because of 'nerves,' so I shouldn't worry, but it was high at home too. I knew that my condition was more serious than the diagnosis said it was."

At Megan's next appointment she discussed her condition in detail with her doctor. As they looked back over her chart and talked about the readings she had gotten at home, it became clear that she needed to go on medication. "I was almost relieved," said Megan. "I didn't really want to be put on medication at such a young age, but I also didn't want to suffer the consequences of not treating my condition."

Since she had planned to start a family soon, Megan made sure she got medication that would be safe for her baby while she was pregnant. "I didn't want to have my body adjust to one medication, then get pregnant and have to switch and adjust again. I figured it would be easier for everyone if I started taking and stayed on the medicine I would take while I was pregnant."

The Nuts and Bolts of Changing Your Life

When it comes to tackling major life changes, the following few techniques are almost universally helpful. Of course, none of these is carved in stone. If you know a better way—something unique that works for you—by all means do it. If not, here are some tried-and-true steps to success.

AIM HIGH: SET PERSONAL GOALS

No matter what lifestyle change you want to make, it generally works best if you break up the process into small, achievable goals. Neither the Taj Mahal nor the Sears Tower was built in a day. Each started as an idea. The architects experimented for months, even years, to design the perfect structure. Along the way, they broke these monumental jobs into small pieces.

Changing your life is no different. Whether you want to lose 50 pounds or complete an hour of physical activity four days a week, making such a change takes lots of little steps over a period of time. Think months—or even years.

You'll need to break up these goals into manageable subgoals. As an example, you might start by formulating an eating plan to lose one to two pounds a week. Every week that you lose at least one pound, give yourself credit for achieving your goal. In a month, you would have lost four to eight pounds. In three months, you may be about halfway to your goal. You might prefer to reward yourself for following your plan for the whole week. Following the plan is under your control; sometimes losing the weight is not.

For this reason, it might work better for you to use your behavior change as the goal rather than the weight loss as the goal.

Goal examples could be:

For two weeks I will eat at least five servings of fruits and vegetables a day and limit my portions of meat, poultry, and seafood to six ounces each day.

OR

I will lose 10 pounds in 12 weeks by walking at least four times each week and by reducing my calorie intake by 300 calories a day.

With the physical activity example, you might start by exercising for 15 minutes a day three days a week. Then you may choose to increase your sessions by five minutes each week until you're exercising for an hour. After a month at this level, you could add an extra day so that you're exercising for one hour four days a week. Both of these scenarios involve breaking the main goal into a series of achievable short-term goals, which add up to reaching your long-term goal. Here are some guidelines:

- *Set challenging but realistic goals.* Seek to lose one to two pounds a week rather than five pounds. One to two pounds is a healthy, realistic weight loss. Five pounds could be unhealthy or unrealistic. One main reason people don't reach their goals is that the goals are not realistic.

- *Set specific, measurable goals.* Rather than setting a goal to improve your upper-body strength, aim to increase the number of push-ups you can do in a single session from 10 to 20. A measurable goal allows you to track the progress you're making.

- *Set short-term goals.* Set goals you can reach within a time period that's short enough to keep you motivated. A goal to lose 35 pounds this year may be too long-range. You might not be able to maintain your focus for a whole year. It's much more reasonable and motivational to set a goal to lose one to two pounds a week for 8 to 12 weeks. You can accomplish that goal, then set a new short-term goal. For most people, it helps to set short-term daily, weekly, and monthly goals that add up over two to three months.

TRACK YOUR GOALS

Setting goals is just the beginning. You'll also want to keep track of your progress. It's okay if your progress is slow, as long as your direction is forward. Tracking your goals is the best way to keep your eye on the prize: the lifestyle change you want to make.

Create a simple goal-tracking sheet. Fill in your long-term goal and set interim goals along the way. Check off your short-term goals as you achieve them, or rework the chart as your needs dictate. Speed is not an issue. Just aim for forward movement toward your goal.

SWEET REWARDS

You also need to keep a list of long- and short-term *rewards*. These rewards are important because they're proof that life can be sweet without overeating and smoking. If you've rewarded yourself in the past by taking a cigarette or cookie break, you'll need to replace those rewards with some that are equally satisfying but more consistent with a healthy lifestyle.

For example, Jeff wanted to increase his physical activity. He set up a three-month plan that added five minutes of physical activity to his daily schedule each week. He planned that by the end of the three months, he'd be doing about an hour a day of moderate physical activity, including mowing the lawn and walking the track with his kids.

Each week that he completed his extra five minutes a day, he rewarded himself. One week, he bought a CD. The next week, he went to a movie. The third week, he took his family on a picnic and hike. When he finally reached his exercise goal of one hour of physical activity a day, he bought himself new running shoes. His reward for sticking with this plan for one year was a family vacation to the Grand Canyon.

The important thing is to make sure your short- and long-term rewards are things that will make you smile. It doesn't matter what the rewards are: attending a concert or sports event, buying clothing, going to the beach, buying a new gadget, launching a creative project, taking a course, going out to dinner at a new place, soaking in a hot tub, or carving out an hour just for yourself. The point is to use these rewards to nurture and motivate yourself. You're worth it.

AVOIDING THE RELAPSE TRAP

On the road to changing your life, the biggest pothole is giving up. You *will* slip up. That's a given. You'll overeat again, you'll sit like a slug for days, you'll sneak a cigarette. It's all part of the process.

This is important enough for us to repeat: A lapse is not failure—it's just a lapse. Failure is when you use a simple slipup as an excuse to quit trying. That's the relapse trap. Fortunately, there's a way out: As soon as you notice the lapse, immediately return to your new, permanent way of living. Go back immediately to eating like a slender person, living like a nonsmoker, exercising like a physically active person. Don't beat yourself up. It's a waste of time. If you have to return 734 times before you become a nonsmoker for life, then do so. Remember, when it comes to changing your life, only one thing is fatal: *giving up.*

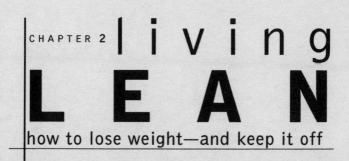

CHAPTER 2 **living**

LEAN

how to lose weight—and keep it off

"GREAT WORKS ARE NOT
PERFORMED BY STRENGTH,
BUT BY PERSEVERANCE."
—SAMUEL JOHNSON

IT'S ALMOST A NATIONAL PLAGUE. SINCE THE LATE 1970S, THE PERCENTAGE OF American women classified as obese has climbed by 21 percent; for men, it's almost 15 percent. Despite a society that worships rail-thin supermodels, many of us struggle along, praying we can still fit into last year's wardrobe and don't have to resort to our "fat clothes."

After you take the Stages of Change Test on page 6, you will know whether you're ready to lose weight. If you're not ready, forget this chapter for now. Instead, focus on where you are in the change process. As you move from stage to stage, you'll eventually be ready to lose your excess weight. On the other hand, if the test shows you're ready, it's time to take a serious look at moving from overweight to a healthy weight.

If you're fighting the battle of the bulge, you have plenty of company. Take a look at the chart that follows. Find your sex and age, and then look at the percentage of your peers who are overweight or obese. Although it's clear that lots of people are trying—and failing—to lose weight, a determined minority are discovering the secrets to losing weight and keeping it off. They've changed their lives, their health, and their self-image for the better.

OVERWEIGHT AMERICANS

AGE	PERCENTAGE OF AMERICANS WHO ARE OVERWEIGHT OR OBESE*
MEN	
20–29	43.1
30–39	58.1
40–49	65.5
50–59	73.0
60–69	70.3
70–79	63.1
80+	50.6
WOMEN	
20–29	33.1
30–39	47.0
40–49	52.7
50–59	64.4
60–69	64.0
70–79	57.9
80+	50.1

SOURCE: The National Heart, Lung, and Blood Institute

* *Among adults 20 to 80+ years, 1988–1994.*

At the American Heart Association, we know these weight-loss secrets. We know that quick weight loss doesn't last and can be unsafe. A loss of one to two pounds a week is safe—and in the long run leads to success. We know what works and what doesn't. In this chapter, we're going to pass these secrets on to you.

How to Keep Your Head While Losing Weight

First of all, relax. You can and will lose weight and change your life, but not by next Saturday's high school reunion. We're talking about a way of life here. That means a new way of eating, thinking, and living.

William James said, "To change one's life: Start immediately. Do it flamboyantly. No exceptions." We think he has the right idea. This is not a "diet"—it's a life exchange. You're permanently turning in your "fat" life for one that's healthier. We'll show you how.

How Does Your Weight Stack Up?

Although getting a true picture of body composition is complex, these simple measurements will help you determine whether yours is in the healthy range.

You'll need a tape measure and a scale. Wear as little as possible and remove your shoes.

1. Measure your waist where it's smallest, usually just above the navel. Breathe out and measure without pulling the tape tight. Record your measurement.

2. Weigh yourself. Record your weight.

3. Stand against a wall and measure your height. Record your height.

WAIST MEASUREMENT

Waist circumference is an indirect way to measure your body composition and risk from overweight. If you're a woman and your waistline measures 35 inches or more, you have a much higher risk for heart disease, stroke, and diabetes. If you're a man, higher risk starts at 40 inches.

BODY MASS INDEX (BMI)

1. Find your height (in inches) along the left side of the BMI chart on pages 40 and 41. Draw a horizontal line across the graph at this height.

2. Find the nearest number to your weight in this row, and draw a vertical line up the graph to the BMI.

3. Read your BMI at the top.

4. Record your BMI.

A BMI of 19 to 24.9 is healthiest—that is, you're at low risk of developing health problems because of your weight. A BMI of 25 to 29.9—considered overweight—carries a moderate risk; 30 and above—considered obese—indicates a high risk. In fact, people with a BMI of 28 or greater are three to four times more likely to have a stroke, heart disease, or diabetes than people with the healthiest BMI.

If your BMI is in the overweight or obese range, look to the left on your height row to see how much weight you need to lose to move down to the healthiest BMI—24. If you're in the obese range now, look at the BMI of 29 and follow the column down to your height row. This will give you an intermediate weight goal, moving from obese to merely overweight. This may make losing weight more doable for you.

For some people, the BMI may not fit the risk categories. For example, muscle weighs more than fat, so bodybuilders may have a higher BMI for their size than the average person. Where health risk is concerned, you have to look at more than weight alone. You must look at *how* your weight is distributed on your body.

Keep a record of your waist measurement, weight, and height. Use these measurements as a baseline to track your improvement. Then weigh yourself and measure your waist again once a month. If you are overweight or obese, your body composition will naturally change for the better when you lose weight. That's especially true if you combine regular physical activity with healthful eating that keeps your weight in the normal range.

BODY MASS INDEX (BMI) CHART

BMI	19	20	21	22	23	24	25	26
HT. (IN.)	BODY WEIGHT (POUNDS)							
58	91	96	100	105	110	115	119	124
59	94	99	104	109	114	119	124	128
60	97	102	107	112	118	123	128	133
61	100	106	111	116	122	127	132	137
62	104	109	115	120	126	131	136	142
63	107	113	118	124	130	135	141	146
64	110	116	122	128	134	140	145	151
65	114	120	126	132	138	144	150	156
66	118	124	130	136	142	148	155	161
67	121	127	134	140	146	153	159	166
68	125	131	138	144	151	158	164	171
69	128	135	142	149	155	162	169	176
70	132	139	146	153	160	167	174	181
71	136	143	150	157	165	172	179	186
72	140	147	154	162	169	177	184	191
73	144	151	159	166	174	182	189	197
74	148	155	163	171	179	186	194	202
75	152	160	168	176	184	192	200	208
76	156	164	172	180	189	197	205	213

27	28	29	30	31	32	33	34	35
			BODY WEIGHT (POUNDS)					
129	134	138	143	148	153	158	162	167
133	138	143	148	153	158	163	168	173
138	143	148	153	158	163	168	174	179
143	148	153	158	164	169	174	180	185
147	153	158	164	169	175	180	186	191
152	158	163	169	175	180	186	191	197
157	163	169	174	180	186	192	197	204
162	168	174	180	186	192	198	204	210
167	173	179	186	192	198	204	210	216
172	178	185	191	198	204	211	217	223
177	184	190	197	203	210	216	223	230
182	189	196	203	209	216	223	230	236
188	195	202	209	216	222	229	236	243
193	200	208	215	222	229	236	243	250
199	206	213	221	228	235	242	250	258
204	212	219	227	235	242	250	257	265
210	218	225	233	241	249	256	264	272
216	224	232	240	248	256	264	272	279
221	230	238	246	254	263	271	279	287

THE HIGH COST OF HEAVYWEIGHTS

If being overweight doesn't seem all that bad, try this: Carry around a 5-pound bag of sugar, a 12-pound turkey, or a 40-pound backpack—all day, *every* day. See how your joints feel; check out your energy level. It's not a great way to live. To make matters worse, excess weight is a major risk factor for heart disease, diabetes, cancer, gallbladder disease, gout, arthritis, breathing problems, and depression.

Eight Great Reasons to Lose Weight

As if looking good in your clothes weren't enough, here are eight eye-opening reasons to shed those extra pounds. Excess weight increases your risk of:

1. CORONARY HEART DISEASE. America's number one killer of both men and women claims about 460,000 lives each year.

2. DIABETES. An epidemic of diabetes, particularly the kind that strikes adults at midlife, has hit the United States. Unless diabetes is carefully regulated, it can lead to heart disease, stroke, kidney disease, blindness, and foot disease.

3. CANCER. The American Cancer Society attributes about one third of the deaths from

cancer to the typical U.S. diet, including its effect on obesity. The cancers most closely linked to obesity include colon, prostate, gall-bladder, breast, uterine, and ovarian.

4. GALLSTONES. Being overweight increases your chances of developing gallstones. More than 500,000 operations are done yearly to correct this painful condition.

5. GOUT. Needlelike crystals of uric acid build up in the joints, causing inflammation, swelling, and pain, especially in the feet. Overeating, especially of protein-rich foods, can cause this type of arthritis.

6. ARTHRITIS. The heavier you are, the more weight you put on your spine, hips, and knees. This weight can wear away cartilage, causing osteoarthritis, which ranges from mild stiffness and aching joints to severe pain and disability.

7. BREATHING PROBLEMS. Excess weight contributes to snoring and sleep apnea, a condition in which breathing stops during sleep. The lack of oxygen wakes you for a brief period, so you start breathing again. At worst, sleep apnea can lead to a heart attack. At best, it interferes with your necessary deep sleep, causing you to wake up in the morning feeling tired. Losing weight reduces the severity of sleep apnea.

8. DEPRESSION. When you're overweight in a culture that worships thinness, you can feel unattractive, ashamed, and depressed, which may cause you to eat more. This cycle can continue spiraling downward into more weight gain and more depression.

OTHER REASONS TO LOSE WEIGHT

Besides these important health problems, you may have other reasons in mind. Check the ones that apply to you.

___I want to feel better.

___I want to look better in my clothes.

___I want to become more physically active so that I can enjoy activities I like.

___I want to be more sexually attractive.

___I want to make a better impression professionally.

___I want to reduce the amount of medication that I take.

___Medical reason: _____

_____

___Other: _____

_____

Write down your top three reasons and post your list on the refrigerator to remind yourself why you are working so hard to lose weight. Also consider your motivation. You may want to lose weight to please others. But people who want to lose weight to achieve their own goals are more likely to succeed at maintaining a long-term weight loss.

WHAT WILL THIS COST?

Now that you know *why* you want to lose weight, you must look realistically at what reaching a healthy weight will cost you. Then figure out whether you're prepared to pay.

Make a list of the costs to you. What will you have to do that you don't do now? What will you have to give up to lose weight? Some costs might be giving up your nightly beer, starting daily walks, or recording your food intake. Others might be giving up the benefits of being overweight: fewer sexual advances to deal with, ability to eat whatever you want, and a ready-made excuse for health problems.

Compare your costs with your list of reasons for losing weight. Do the pros of losing weight outweigh the cons? If not, stop reading here. If they do, let's look at the challenges ahead.

Preparing to Face the Challenges

You've already decided that you can change your eating and your activity behaviors. Now consider the strength of your desire to lose weight.

Have you decided to lose weight?
__Yes __No

Will you follow your program for three months?
__Yes __No

Thinking about work and your personal life, is this the right time to start a weight-loss program?
__Yes __No

Will you be happy with a weight loss of one to two pounds per week?
__Yes __No

If your answer to all four questions is yes, let's proceed to the specific challenges you may face.

CHALLENGE CHECKLIST

Check the challenges that may be a problem for you.

__Seeing food

__Having tempting foods at home

__Feeling depressed or angry

__Going to a party

__Celebrating

__Eating out

__Brisk walking or doing a similar activity for at least 30 minutes

__Exercising at least three days a week

__Other _____

For every challenge, come up with a plan of action that will help you move past it—and keep you moving in the direction of your new healthful lifestyle.

Seeing food. Keep food packages out of sight in the pantry. Put raw vegetables and fruits in front in the refrigerator so that's what you see first. Order your groceries online so you're not walking through the supermarket seeing a lot of tempting foods to put in the basket.

Having tempting foods at home. Instead of bringing home a half gallon of ice cream, have one scoop when you're out.

Feeling depressed or angry. Take a walk or call a friend and talk.

Going to a party. Plan what you will do at the party other than eat. Talk to at least five people. Take pictures. Keep a glass of water or diet soda in one hand.

Celebrating. Think of an activity other than eating. Go to a movie (skip their popcorn). Spend a couple of hours at the zoo or the botanic gardens.

Exercising. See the physical activity chapter, page 115.

jim's story:
WHO'S IN CHARGE HERE?

"I've been fighting overweight all my life," remembered Jim, a 52-year-old graphic designer. "To my mom, food was love. She had food for every situation. When I got home from school, she had warm cookies and milk for me. I was always a fat kid. I was miserable being teased all the time, but Mom thought food would cure anything. She stood over me until I cleaned my plate. At college, I tried to diet on my own. In fact, I'd starve myself for days, not eat anything, then binge like crazy.

"After I married, I thought it would be easier," said Jim. "I thought I would lose weight and live normally. But something always got in the way, and I kept postponing really losing."

Jim ate if he had a bad day at work. He ate to celebrate his wife's birthday. If they had an argument, he ate.

One day, standing in front of the refrigerator looking for his favorite—chocolate chocolate-chip ice cream—Jim realized that food controlled his life. He knew he would have to learn to manage his emotions and his eating.

He found nutrition information on the Internet and created an eating plan that included no "dieting." Instead, it had three healthful meals a day, with protein, vegetables, fruits, and whole grains. He also added some nutritious snacks and an occasional beer. Twice a month he allowed himself a high-calorie dessert.

"I knew I had to get control of this weight problem, or it was going to control me for the rest of my life," said Jim. "There were a few false starts, but finally I adopted this healthier way of eating. My wife was getting interested in health too, so she helped me with the menus and the cooking. I also did a lot of work on my emotions and how to handle them. Today, I'm just a couple of pounds above a normal weight. I maintain it with this same way of eating. I also started running and lifting weights at the Y. I'm glad I'm now in control of my weight and my life. It feels good."

MAKING YOUR GENES FIT

It may be tempting to believe that you inherited your tendency to gain weight. After all, some people seem naturally thin, others naturally hefty. In reality, genes account for only 25 to 40 percent of your weight-gaining tendencies; environment accounts for 60 to

75 percent. For most people, the amount of food you eat and the physical activity you engage in have a much more powerful effect on your weight than heredity has. The following simple equations explain the correlation between calories, physical activity, and weight. Weight gain is a simple equation:

IF NUMBER OF CALORIES YOU EAT	*EQUALS*	NUMBER OF CALORIES YOU BURN IN ACTIVITY, YOUR WEIGHT STAYS THE SAME.
IF NUMBER OF CALORIES YOU EAT	*IS GREATER THAN*	NUMBER OF CALORIES YOU BURN IN ACTIVITY, YOU GAIN WEIGHT.
IF NUMBER OF CALORIES YOU EAT	*IS LESS THAN*	NUMBER OF CALORIES YOU BURN IN ACTIVITY, YOU LOSE WEIGHT.

No matter what diet you try, this calories-in/calories-out equation is inescapable. That's good news because it means you have all the control—if you want it. You can choose what to eat and what not to eat, when to boost your physical activity level, and when to get some R and R. You call the shots.

NEVER SAY DIET

If you study the people who lose weight and keep it off, they'll tell you that they're not following a diet. Dieting means eating a special way to lose weight, then going back to eating "normally." At the American Heart Association, we know that losing weight and keeping it off involves a total lifestyle change— not simply following a diet.

Obesity experts agree that fad diets don't work. That's because they're often bizarre eating plans that no one can follow for more than a few months. Then the dieter returns to his or her "regular food," also returning to his or her former weight. Just remember: No magical diets or miracle foods will make you skinny. Neither will secret formulas, food combinations, or miracle pills. There is only living the life of a fat person or living the life of a slender person. You choose.

Ten Secrets to Losing Weight— and Keeping It Off

Nothing will change your life quite like losing weight. You're treated differently at 250 pounds than you are at 150 pounds. People respond differently to overweight people than they do to healthy-weight people. It may not be fair, but that's the way it is. You feel, look, and act different too. Your entire life— from your relationships, the foods you eat, and the clothes you wear to the activities you engage in— changes when you lose weight. Even your view of yourself changes.

People who manage this transition successfully have learned the following 10 secrets to life-changing weight loss. In their move from overweight to a healthy weight, these people have taken each of the issues to heart, making them part of who they are. Now it's your turn. You can make a fresh start.

1. REFRIGERATOR PHOTO—SEE YOURSELF AS ALREADY SLENDER

If you've been overweight for a long time, it's difficult to see yourself as anything but heavy. It's easy to believe the doom-and-gloom folks who claim that once heavy, always heavy. Before you can lose weight, you need to look carefully at these myths, then change your perception of what is possible for you.

FACTS AND FALLACIES

You may have heard people make the following claims often—so often, in fact, that you may actually *believe* them. People say:

- If you've tried to lose weight many times and haven't reached your ideal weight, you will never succeed. *Wrong!*

- You can't ever eat anything good again. *Wrong!*

- You have to exercise 24 hours a day. *Wrong!*

- You'll never be able to do it on your own. *Wrong!*

- You'll hit a weight plateau and stay there forever. *Wrong!*

- Even if you lose weight, you'll eventually gain it all back. *Wrong!*

All these statements are *wrong!* People like you prove them false every day. Take a look at the facts.

- In one group of people who've lost weight and kept it off for at least three years—"good losers"—about 45 percent were overweight as children and teenagers. Being heavy most of your life doesn't mean you have to stay that way.

- Almost 60 percent of these good losers tried to lose weight at least five times before they were successful. Another 20 percent tried three or four times before winning the battle of the bulge. If you've tried before, you have experience to draw on.

- Good losers don't starve themselves. They eat three average meals a day, plus snacks, or five or six small meals. They don't deny themselves any foods, including sweets. They eat whatever they want, but in moderation. For example, people who have lost weight may still treat themselves to a piece of cake or pie for dessert, but they have a smaller piece than they used to eat, and they indulge only once or twice a week.

- As for exercise, about 70 percent of these good losers exercise three or more times a week, usually walking. Although they're more active than the general population, they're not superjocks.

- Age doesn't matter. Some good losers drop 50 or more pounds in their 60s or 70s. You can lose weight at a safe, reasonable speed *at any age* if you coordinate your calorie intake with your activity output.

- About half the good losers lost weight on their own; the other half did so with the help of a support program. Virtually all maintain their weight loss without group support.

- Plateaus are only temporary. Although people do hit plateaus, sometimes long ones, they will move on to lose their remaining excess weight if they permanently change their way of eating and exercising.

- Although it's great to have an ambitious weight goal, about one-third of good losers settle for a maintenance weight that's somewhat higher than their original goal. For example, a man who's 5 feet 8 inches tall and weighs 240 pounds may want to reach 160. When he gets to that point, however, he may find that it's too difficult to maintain, so he settles for a still healthy—but easier to maintain—180 to 185 pounds.

BELIEVE IN YOURSELF

A study of people who lost weight and kept it off reported that they had started believing in themselves as the ultimate authority. They had all taken a long look at themselves and found an inner determination that they could maintain a thin body and had "no need to return to a heavy one."

Just as you may want to blame heredity, it may be tempting to feel that your overweight condition is the result of fate. As the stories in this section show, however, your weight is completely within your control. People who've been successful at losing weight describe moving from a state of hopelessness to one of self-control and power.

Although we at the American Heart Association firmly believe in attaining and maintaining a healthy weight for the health benefits, we know that you may want to lose weight only to look better. The next few pages focus on that aspect of weight loss, but the ideas apply equally well to weight loss that makes you feel better and helps prevent disease.

daniel's story:
IMAGINE YOURSELF THIN

"I've always been a little overweight and shy, a little unsure of myself. That's why after I graduated from college, I just concentrated on work. I was in the library or at the computer twenty-four hours a day, it seemed," said Daniel, a technical writer.

"I began to gain more weight. Then it became a vicious cycle: I'd gain weight, be depressed and ashamed, isolate myself even more, eat more, and gain more weight. I felt powerless to stop this process."

By age 26, Daniel had ballooned to more than 200 pounds. He did nothing but work, play computer games, and sleep. He was miserable, but didn't know what to do to change that.

"During this time, I had a coworker who went on a diet and lost sixty pounds. What a change, not only in her looks, but in her personality. She was dramatically happier. And I knew this girl. She was not a superbrain or anything. I decided if *she* could do it, I could do it."

Daniel started thinking of creating a new, thinner, happier, in-control self. He started with the same diet his coworker used, but quickly modified it to suit his weight and eating style. He ate a moderate amount of protein, plenty of fruits and vegetables, and healthful snacks. He learned to make great stir-fry dinners. As his weight began to drop, Daniel felt a surge of confidence, so he joined a Tae Bo class. At first, he stayed in the back of the classroom, but as his weight came off and his muscle tone improved, he moved toward the front.

"Today, I'm a new person," said Daniel. "I can hardly remember that guy who lived at the computer and ate his way through life. I work, but not all the time. I eat normally and even treat myself to the occasional wild splurge, but I'm busy and involved in life. I have new friends and activities. I joined the office softball team and started working out at the gym. I just see myself in a new light. Food is no longer in control—I am."

There are thousands of stories like Daniel's. In these stories, the people caught a new vision of themselves as powerful, in-control individuals who could recast themselves in life as permanently slender. In short, they knew they could do it, so they did.

2. DO IT FOR *YOU*

Cathy's husband, Bill, is constantly after her to lose weight. When he's around, he monitors every bite of food she eats. He chides her when she overindulges. When Bill is watching, Cathy eats healthful, balanced meals, fully intending to lose weight; but when he leaves, she binges on junk food. He can't understand why she isn't losing weight. She feels guilty for sabotaging her weight-loss efforts.

This scenario is doomed to fail for one simple reason: The heavy person is not in control. She's not trying to lose weight for *herself*—she's making an attempt to please someone else. Every day, this scenario is repeated between parents and overweight children, between spouses or best friends, between coaches and players, or in any other relationship where one person is pushing another to lose weight.

If you're in a situation where someone wants you to lose weight more than you do, the result will be sheer disaster—unless you set a boundary and take control for yourself. The choice to lose weight or stay heavy is *yours and yours alone.*

If you don't want to lose weight, your job is to accept and love yourself just as you are. Tell the other person—let's say it's your sister—that although you appreciate her interest, your size is your choice. Tell her you like the way you are. Explain that her job is to handle her own life and happiness; your job is to handle your own life and happiness—including your size. Get your sister's promise to support your decision, and get her to let go of trying to change you.

If you *do* want to lose weight, your job is to thank your sister for her interest, but explain that you intend to lose weight in *your* way, at *your* pace, and in *your* own time. Tell her that her job is to support you in whatever you want to do—and nothing else. Then take control of your weight-loss efforts and completely call the shots. *You* decide everything: when, how, and how much. If your sister tries to take back control of the situation, gently but firmly explain that she should concentrate on herself and leave your decisions (and actions) to you. Then make what you said stick.

LOVE THYSELF

Decide to lose excess weight because you *are* a wonderful person, not to become one.

linda's story:
"SHE'S SO PRETTY"

"All my life, my mother, teachers, and friends would try to get me to lose weight. Their feeling about me was, 'She's so pretty; it's too bad she's fat,'" Linda explained. "My mother was especially concerned about my weight. She said that boys didn't like fat girls."

Eventually Linda fell in love with one of the few men who seemed not to care about her weight. They married. In the security of feeling loved for herself, Linda decided to lose weight. The following January, she joined a weight-loss program during its New Year's promotion special. It wasn't easy, but by using the eating plan with nutritionally balanced meals and plenty of snacks, she was able to retrain herself about food. For activity, she chose walking as a start. She asked her husband to support her by walking with her. He got up early so they could walk before work. He did exactly what she asked him to do and never criticized her food choices. "This was the kind of support I needed," said Linda.

The first six months, she lost 32 pounds. Then she lost about three pounds a month until she got down to her goal weight of 140. "This is a comfortable weight for me to maintain, walking five days a week and going to yoga class one evening a week. I also allow myself ice cream once a week as a treat. I can do this for the rest of my life," she said.

GET A (NEW LEASE ON) LIFE

Studies of people who have lost weight permanently show that finally losing weight and keeping it off was not the result of a single decision. It was the result of multiple changes, such as the ones that follow. If you plan to lose weight and keep it off, work on incorporating some of the same ideas into your life.

- *Put yourself first.* Develop a kind of selfishness about your weight. As one good loser said, "I got ornery. I got stubborn. I figured out what it takes to take care of myself and did it."

- *Discover the "payoff" to being fat.* Find out what not losing weight does for you. Does it allow you to hide? Avoid intimacy? Escape dealing with sexual attraction? If you can't see what the payoff is, work with a professional counselor until you do.

- *Realize that it's not all that easy being thin, either.* Although being a healthy weight has a massive upside, it has a downside too. People's expectations of you, the cost of buying new clothing, resentful friends, too much praise for your weight loss, problems from the past that losing weight won't solve—you'll have to deal with all of them, so get prepared.

- *Anticipate the positive.* In addition to challenges, be aware of and prepared to handle positive changes. Shopping with more choices of clothes, no "fat" discrimination, improved health and energy, and liking yourself and your new looks are all "good stresses."

- *Realize that losing weight will never be easy.* Losing weight is hard. Period. And it's not fair that you need to lose weight. You can choose to accept the situation and work hard, or you can give up. The choice is yours.

- *Realize that you won't always be motivated.* When you first start losing weight and get lots of compliments, it's easy to stay motivated. When you're in maintenance mode or you've hit a plateau, though, it's tough. It helps to realize that sometimes you'll be motivated, but other times you won't. Stick with your new lifestyle over time the best you can.

- *Sometimes you'll fail, and that's okay.* You'll backslide, trust us. Failure is actually a part of weight-loss success. If you relapse and begin to overeat, catch yourself, admit that it's only a step in the process, and go back to your new, permanent way of eating. No recriminations, no guilt. Simply return.

- *Heads up—maintenance is an active stance.* Your new slender lifestyle is a way of life—an active way of life. That means you constantly seek new solutions to overeating. Be creative and proactive. Any problem has many solutions. Find yours.

- *No rush.* Take your time. This is not a race. Lose weight gradually at a safe, grounded pace. You're more likely to keep it off that way.

3. THERE'S ONLY ONE WAY TO LOSE WEIGHT: *YOURS*

We have good news and bad news. The bad news is that we have no miracle weight-loss diet for you to follow. The good news is *the same thing*. Ask people who've permanently lost weight how they did it, and they'll all tell you something different. The bottom line? Find something that works for you, and then do it.

Most people who have mastered weight loss eventually settle into a way of eating that includes lots of fruits, vegetables, whole-grain foods, and nonfat and low-fat dairy foods; a modest amount of protein; and a low to moderate amount of fat. They even splurge on high-fat, high-calorie foods occasionally. In fact, no food is taboo . . . just eat in moderation.

The overall idea is that as long as it's safe and healthful, *you* choose the way you want to lose weight. Only you know what will work for you. Everyone is wired differently.

kendrick's story:
A MIND OF HIS OWN

"I've never done anything like anybody else," said Kendrick, "and I'm not going to start now." He always loved to eat, but when he found himself 55 pounds overweight, he decided he had to do something.

"I wasn't going to join some weight-loss group, that's for sure," he said. "What I did was come up with my own diet. I'm a lineman for the phone company, so I ate a big breakfast for lots of energy, a regular lunch, and a small supper. Mainly, I just pushed back from the table sooner. I also cut back on sodas and switched from regular to diet drinks. I'd been drinking a liter of pop a day.

"The danger point for me is at night. I crave sweets and snack foods between 8:00 and 10:00." Kendrick substituted fruit, low-fat popcorn, and pretzels for high-fat snacks. He also joined a basketball team that had its practice games on Monday and Wednesday nights, with the actual games on the weekend. This served two purposes: The activity burned calories, and it kept him busy during his most tempting eating period.

Kendrick's weight-loss strategies have worked. He's almost at his goal weight, and he plans to modify his new way of eating, keep up his sport, and continue his new lifestyle indefinitely.

DO-IT-YOURSELF WEIGHT LOSS

According to good losers, about half of them did it with eating plans they designed themselves; the other half did it through organized programs. Almost none of them lost weight and kept it off by following a fad diet or by taking diet pills.

When asked how they finally permanently lost weight, the people who made up their own programs explained:

- "I threw out the scale and changed my daily activities and attitudes about food."

- "Eating tiny meals and lots of willpower."

- "Regular exercise, eating low-fat healthy foods, and eating only when hungry."

- "Watched my diet closely and exercised. No seconds at meals, no bread, no soft drinks and sweets. Plus I had a friend do it with me, and we gave each other encouragement."

The organized-program people used the program for their initial weight loss, but maintained their new weight on their own.

Although each camp can claim many successes, studies show that people who create their own eating plan are more likely to maintain weight loss over time. Another secret to their success is splurging occasionally with their favorite foods so they don't feel deprived. The people who followed a program successfully found a way to customize the program to their specifications. In short, they made it their own.

By contrast, people who took diet pills, fasted, did hypnosis, participated in fad diets, and strictly denied themselves the foods they loved almost always regained their lost weight.

REMEMBER THE TURTLE

Slow and steady wins the race. If you start on January 1 and lose just one pound a week this year by eating in your new, permanent, healthful way, you'll be 52 pounds lighter on December 31.

WHAT WORKS FOR YOU?

If you've tried to lose weight before and failed, you probably know what works for you and what doesn't. Write down a list of habits and ideas that worked, along with those that failed. List the foods and calorie levels that worked best, the amount of restriction, how you prepared the food and shopped, how you felt both mentally and physically, what exercise worked best, what was difficult, what was easy, and how you modified your daily routine to help you reach your goal. Then style your own eating plan from the ideas that worked. For example:

WHAT WORKED	WHAT DIDN'T WORK
Eating five smaller meals a day	Skipping lunch
Eating your favorite foods occasionally	Strict dieting
Packing your lunch the night before	Eating grapefruit five times a day
Limiting alcohol	Drinking nothing but water
Brisk walking four times a week	Strict, heavy exercise schedule

If you decide to join a weight-loss program, watch out for plans that:

- Overemphasize one food or food group (unbalanced, dangerous)

- Say you can eat all you want and still lose weight (impossible)

- Guarantee results (again, impossible)

- Claim that curing allergies will help you lose weight (overeating, not allergies, causes overweight)

- Offer foods that burn fat (no known food or combination of foods burns fat)

- Offer body wraps, injections, herbs, and cellulite treatments (results are not permanent)

- Promise breakthrough findings or weight-loss secrets of the ages (if these existed, they'd make front-page news everywhere)

- Advocate eating less than 1,200 calories a day (nutritionally inadequate, even with vitamins)

- Tout surgery or drugs (be aware of potential risks)

4. YOU ARE WHAT YOU EAT— REALLY!

You want to lose weight. You want to be healthy, be slender, wear attractive clothes, and never be concerned about being overweight again. No problem. You can do it. All you have to do is eat like slender people eat.

Actually, many slender people eat a lot. But they eat a lot of the right things. They've discovered a way of eating that lets them fill up without ballooning up. They understand one simple fact: *You are what you eat.* If you eat fried foods, butter-drenched cream sauces, candy, and entire cheesecakes, you're going to look like it. If you eat fruits, vegetables, protein, whole-grain foods, and nonfat and low-fat dairy foods and splurge only now and then, you're going to look like that. It's a choice that has consequences.

Given that fact, you can easily decide which lifestyle you want to adopt—an overweight lifestyle or a normal-weight lifestyle. The weight follows the lifestyle. If you choose the normal-weight lifestyle, keep reading. We'll show you the joys of eating without guilt, recrimination, and struggle. We'll offer some tips and guidelines to help you create an eating plan you can lose weight on—and live with—for life.

PICK AND CHOOSE YOUR CALORIES

Some foods are packed with vital nutrients. Some give you only calories. For example, although a calorie is a calorie as far as weight is concerned, 100 calories' worth of pie doesn't translate in your body the same way as 100 calories' worth of broccoli. That's because one of these foods contains many calories from sugar and fat, and most of the calories in the other come from complex carbohydrate packed with vitamins, minerals, and fiber. The 100 calories from pie come from about a third of an average slice; the 100 calories from broccoli fill an entire plate. If you have 100 calories to spend, consider that your body will be better off with more vitamins, minerals, and fiber than with more sugar and fat. Try to spend your calories well. Think of it as getting the biggest bang for your buck!

Basically, food comes in three categories: protein, carbohydrate, and fat. It pays to know how each affects your health and weight. It also pays to get the best nutrition bargain you can for the calories that you put into your mouth. Each category is important for good health, so remember to eat a variety of foods with a variety of nutrients.

Protein

Meats, seafood, poultry, dairy foods, and eggs all furnish complete protein. This means they provide all the amino acids your body needs. In this country, it has become routine to eat lots of protein—we can afford it! However, you need only five to six ounces of complete protein a day to meet your nutritional needs.

It's best to have two servings a day of two and a half to three ounces each (cooked weight). A three-ounce serving of cooked meat, poultry, or fish is about the size of a deck of cards. This is not your typical steak-house serving, which is frequently seven to nine ounces cooked.

Another good source of protein is fat-free and low-fat dairy products. In addition to protein, they furnish healthy amounts of calcium, which you need to keep your bones strong.

Except for protein from soybeans and quinoa (a South American grain), plant proteins are not complete. You can get complete protein by combining legumes (peas and beans) with grains (such as whole-grain bread, corn, and oats). You don't even have to eat them in the same meal—just on the same day.

Compared to fat, protein offers a bargain in calories. Each gram of protein contains only four calories, but fat contains nine calories per gram. Much animal protein, such as marbled steaks and most sausage, is interwoven with high-calorie fat. Choose your protein wisely to save calories.

Carbohydrates

Carbohydrates, which also contain four calories per gram, come in two varieties: simple and complex. Simple carbohydrates include sugars, such as granulated sugar, corn syrup, and honey, which are used in sweets of all kinds. Fruits also are a source of simple carbohydrates, including the sugar fructose, but fruits are good for you because they are rich in vitamins and minerals. Good sources of complex carbohydrates, such as vegetables and whole grains, provide fiber as well as vitamins and minerals. In general, the less processing that has gone into fruits, vegetables, and grains, the more healthful they are.

Some people claim that carbohydrates such as breads and potatoes are bad for you. Actually, it's the spreads and sauces slathered on these foods that cause the health problem. Plain bread, especially whole-wheat and other whole-grain bread, is good for you. A plain baked or boiled potato gives you a lot of nutrients, including fiber and vitamin C.

Okay, so you don't want to eat bread or potatoes plain. Try all-fruit spread, tub or spray margarine, nonfat sour cream, butter-flavor sprinkles, low-fat salsa . . . or come up with your own low-fat, low-calorie spread or sauce. Just don't write off bread and potatoes as fattening.

Fats

At a price of nine calories per gram, fats really make you splurge in calories. To help reduce your calorie intake, try to keep your total fat intake below 30 percent of calories. Don't just focus on fat, though. You can't eat nonfat and low-fat baked goods as though there's no tomorrow and expect to consume a reasonable number of calories.

The American Heart Association recommends that less than 10 percent of your total calories should come from saturated fat. If you're on a 1,500-calorie-a-day plan, that makes your limit of saturated fat about 17 grams a day.

An eating plan relatively low in saturated fat and cholesterol helps protect you against heart disease. This is true whether you're overweight or not.

Saturated Fats

These raise LDL cholesterol in your blood. LDL is known as the "bad" cholesterol carrier because it deposits cholesterol on artery walls. You'll find saturated fat mainly in foods of animal origin, such as meats, poultry, lard, butter, and whole-milk dairy products. You'll also find it in coconuts, coconut oil, palm and palm kernel oil, and cocoa butter. Vegetable sources of saturated fat are often found in commercially baked goods, so be on the lookout. Read the labels on prepared foods to find the amount of saturated fat in a serving. Choose products that are lower in saturated fat to help you stay within your limit.

Trans Fats

These fats also raise your cholesterol. When poly-unsaturated vegetable oils are hardened into margarine and other shortenings, they become partially hydrogenated oils, containing trans fat. Research has linked this fat to heart disease. Although a little bit won't hurt, you'll want to limit foods containing trans fats. Trans fats are found in fast foods such as french fries and doughnuts; packaged cookies, cakes, and crackers; and some stick margarines. Liquid and tub (or soft) margarines contain almost no trans fats. They are your best choice. Read product labels for "hydrogenated" or "partially hydrogenated," and limit the amount of these foods you eat.

Dietary Cholesterol

This can also raise the level of cholesterol in your blood, increasing the risk of heart attack. You get cholesterol in two ways: Your body manufactures all you need, and you get some from foods. Cholesterol comes only from foods of animal origin, such as egg yolks, meats, seafood, poultry, and dairy products. We recommend keeping your dietary cholesterol intake to less than 300 milligrams a day; it should be less than 200 milligrams per day if you have had a heart attack or have high cholesterol.

Polyunsaturated and Monounsaturated Fats

These fats may help reduce the amount of cholesterol in your blood when you use them in place of saturated fats. You'll find omega-3 polyunsaturated fat in certain kinds of fish, such as salmon, haddock, and sardines, and in flaxseed oil. Foods high in mono-unsaturated fats include olive oil, canola oil, peanut oil, avocados, walnuts, and almonds.

WHAT TO EAT

Okay, it's time to create your own personal eating plan. Although no foods are forbidden, it helps to understand which kinds and amounts of food promote health and weight loss and which do not. At the American Heart Association, we believe that our Healthy Heart Food Pyramid is a great guideline for healthy eating.

Take a look. We simply fit all foods into this pyramid in rough proportion to how much of each kind you should eat to be healthy and lose weight. For example, it's easy to see that most of the pyramid—the wider parts at the bottom—consists of two food groups: breads, cereals, pasta, and starchy vegetables are in one, and fruits and vegetables make up the other. When you're planning what to eat every day, take most of your food from these groups. They're low in fat and calories and high in nutrition.

Continuing up the pyramid, you'll find the next two food groups: fat-free milk and low-fat dairy products in one, and lean meat, poultry, and seafood

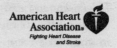
Healthy Heart
Food Pyramid

Fats, oils, nuts & sweets
Use sparingly

Fat-free milk, low-fat
dairy products
2-4 per day

Lean meat, poultry and seafood
**No more than 6 oz.
(cooked) per day**

Vegetables & fruits
5 or more per day

Breads, cereals,
pasta & starchy
vegetables
**6 or more
per day**

- The American Heart Association has adapted the Food Guide Pyramid, developed by the U.S. Dept. of Agriculture and U.S. Dept. of Health and Human Services, to be consistent with the AHA Dietary Guidelines for Healthy American Adults.
- Beans and potatoes are included with starchy vegetables.
- Limit your sodium intake to no more than 3,000 milligrams per day.
- Eat no more than 3-4 egg yolks per week. (Egg whites are not limited.)
- For more information, call your local AHA office or 1-800-AHA-USA1 (1-800-242-8721) and ask for the "American Heart Association Diet: An Eating Plan for Healthy Americans" or "Easy Food Tips for Heart-Healthy Eating."

©1994, 1996, American Heart Association

in the other. These foods contain protein, calcium, and a host of other nutrients. Notice that they take up less space in the pyramid—which means they should take up less space in your eating plan.

At the very top of the pyramid, you'll find foods you'll want to monitor carefully. These are fats, oils, nuts, and sweets. This group includes high-fat processed foods, such as potato chips and candy. Because this food group contains by far the most fat and calories, you'll want to skimp here. While you're losing weight, you may want to drastically restrict the foods in this part of the pyramid. After you've lost the weight, you can begin to include them in your eating plan in a small way.

For example, Louise decided to get serious about changing the unhealthful way she ate. She eliminated all high-fat snacks, fried foods, and desserts from her eating plan. She lost 21 pounds in just three months. After she reached her goal weight, she decided to add two high-fat snacks (she loves almonds) and two desserts to her weekly eating plan. To help burn calories, she continues her three-mile walks four days a week. After more than two years, Louise is still at her goal weight. As for fried foods, she lost her taste for them. Now she prefers broiled or grilled foods.

Feel free to use this pyramid to create an eating plan that works for you. Take into consideration your caloric needs, your work schedule, your activities, your hungriest times of the day, the need for healthful snacks, and times you are likely to binge. Build an eating plan that offers new and creative solutions to old problems.

Allow yourself some wiggle room. You don't have to lose all your excess weight by next Thursday. Go at a pace that's safe and right for you. After all, this way of eating is not a "diet." It's the normal way you'll be eating for life, continually adjusting it to keep your health good, your body slender, and the good times rolling. Because this way of eating will last a lifetime, you'll have a lifetime to enjoy it. There's no rush.

QUANTITY

We don't want to get too picky here. It's your eating plan, so you create it. But a word to the wise: Watch your serving sizes. For example, in the average Italian restaurant, you get a brimming bowl of pasta. Whoa, there. A normal serving of pasta is about one-half cup. The jumbo bagels at the grocery store look normal, but they're two or three times as big as an average serving of bread. A steak the size of a plate should feed six people, not one.

If you're still hungry after eating realistic servings, eat more salad, vegetables, beans, and other high-fiber, high-nutrition foods. You'll see results faster.

Below is a quick overview of the food groups, along with the number of recommended servings and serving sizes the average person needs every day. If you've been overeating, the guidelines are a good way to see normal eating at a glance.

Breads, cereals, pasta, and starchy vegetables

About six servings a day for adults; four for children and preteens. A serving size is:

1 slice bread
⅓ to ½ bagel
½ cup cooked pasta
1 cup flaked cereal
½ cup nugget-type cereal
½ cup cooked cereal
¼ to ½ cup starchy vegetables, such as potatoes

Vegetables and fruits

At least five servings a day. A serving size is:

1 medium piece of fruit
½ to 1 cup cooked or raw vegetables or fruit
½ cup fruit or vegetable juice

Fat-free milk and nonfat or low-fat dairy products

Two servings a day for most people; four servings a day for teens and pregnant or breast-feeding women; and three servings a day for people over 65. A serving size is:

1 cup fat-free milk
1 cup nonfat or low-fat yogurt
1 ounce nonfat or low-fat cheese
½ cup nonfat or low-fat cottage cheese

Lean meat, poultry, seafood, and eggs

Two servings a day. A serving size is:

4 ounces raw lean meat (3 ounces cooked)
4 ounces raw poultry (3 ounces cooked)
4 ounces raw seafood (3 ounces cooked)

Eggs need special mention because of the high cholesterol content of the yolks. One serving includes only one egg yolk, with no more than one yolk per day. On days that you eat an egg yolk, you need to carefully monitor other cholesterol-containing foods to stay under 300 milligrams of cholesterol for the day.

You may choose to use egg substitute or egg whites for egg yolks. Two egg whites equal one egg.

Fats, oils, nuts, and sweets

Five to eight servings a day, depending on your caloric needs. Limit yourself to five a day if you're trying to lose weight. A serving size is:

1 teaspoon vegetable oil
1 teaspoon margarine, with no more than 2 grams of saturated fat per tablespoon
2 teaspoons diet margarine
1 tablespoon chopped nuts
1 tablespoon seeds without shells
1 tablespoon salad dressing
2 teaspoons mayonnaise
2 teaspoons peanut butter
10 small or 5 large olives

⅛ medium avocado

1½ tablespoons sugar, syrup, jam, honey, or preserves

6 fluid ounces lemonade or sweetened carbonated beverage

¾ ounce candy made primarily with sugar, such as gum-
drops, mints, and hard candies

1 slice angel food cake (¹⁄₂₄ of a cake)

2 gingersnaps

⅓ cup fruit ice or sherbet

½ cup fruit-flavored gelatin

1 fig bar cookie

SHOPPING

No matter what eating plan you've created, you'll need some low-fat, low-calorie, high-nutrition basics. Fill your refrigerator and pantry with foods designed to help you lose weight and keep it off. These foods include:

Fat-free or low-fat milk, yogurt, cheese, and cottage cheese

Light or diet margarine

Egg or egg substitute

Sandwich breads, bagels, pita bread, and English muffins

Soft corn tortillas and low-fat flour tortillas

Plain cereal, dry or hot

Rice

Pasta

White-meat chicken and turkey (don't eat the skin)

Fish and shellfish (not battered)

Beef: round, sirloin, chuck arm, loin, and extra-lean-ground beef

Pork: leg, shoulder, and tenderloin
Dried beans and peas
Fresh, frozen, and canned fruits without added sugar
Fresh, frozen, or no-salt-added canned vegetables
Fat-free or low-fat salad dressings
Mustard and ketchup
All-fruit spread
Herbs and spices
Nonfat salsa

PREPARED FOODS

You can control the amount of fat and calories you eat when you buy and cook for yourself. But what about prepared foods? All you need to do is read the nutrition label on the package. There you'll find the serving size; the number of calories per serving; and the amounts of total fat, saturated fat, and cholesterol in a single serving.

As the sample nutrition label that follows on page 82 shows, you can determine how much fat and how many calories you're getting in a serving of that food. Choose foods that are lower in fat. Eating to lose weight is easy—just read the labels and it all adds up.

Grocery guide to food labels

Thanks to the Food and Drug Administration (FDA), food manufacturers are required to meet strict criteria for the nutrition claims they put on their foods. The claims and what they mean are on page 83.

Nutrition Facts

Serving Size 1/2 cup (114g)
Servings Per Container 4

Amount Per Serving

Calories 90   Calories from Fat 30

% Daily Value*

Total Fat 3g	**5%**
Saturated Fat 0g	**0%**
Cholesterol 0mg	**0%**
Sodium 300mg	**13%**
Total Carbohydrate 13g	**4%**
Dietary Fiber 3g	**12%**
Sugars 3g	
Protein 3g	

Vitamin A	80%	• Vitamin C	60%
Calcium	4%	• Iron	4%

*Percent Daily Values are based on a 2,000
calorie diet. Your daily values may be higher or
lower depending on your calorie needs:

	Calories	2,000	2,500
Total Fat	Less than	65g	80g
Sat. Fat	Less than	20g	25g
Cholesterol	Less than	300mg	300mg
Sodium	Less than	2,400mg	2,400mg
Total Carbohydrate		300g	375g
Fiber		25g	30g

Calories per gram:
Fat 9   •   Carbohydrate 4   •   Protein 4

CLAIM	DEFINITION
Fat free	Less than 0.5 g of fat per serving
Low fat	3 g of fat or less per serving
Reduced or less fat	At least 25 percent less saturated fat than the regular version of this food
Cholesterol free	Less than 2 mg of cholesterol and 2 g or less of saturated fat per serving
Low cholesterol	20 mg or less and 2 g or less of saturated fat per serving
Reduced or less cholesterol	At least 25 percent less than the regular version and 2 g or less of saturated fat per serving
Sodium free	Less than 5 mg of sodium per serving
Low sodium	140 mg or less of sodium per serving
Reduced or less sodium	At least 25 percent less sodium per serving than the regular version
Very low sodium	35 mg or less of sodium per serving
High fiber	5 g or more of fiber per serving
Good source of fiber	2.5 to 4.9 g of fiber per serving
More or added fiber	At least 2.5 g more of fiber per serving than the regular food

You'll find that some food labels boast a heart with a check mark through it. This means that the food meets the American Heart Association criteria for

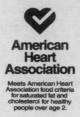

saturated fat and cholesterol levels for healthy people over age two. When you see this symbol, you know you're buying a heart-smart product.

ADAPTING RECIPES

It's no state secret. Some cooking methods add lots of fat and calories to foods, and others do not. For example, fried chicken is loaded with fat; broiled chicken without the skin is not. Vegetables cooked with bacon have added calories and saturated fat; steamed vegetables do not. That's why you'll want to find low-fat, low-cal ways of cooking your favorite foods.

To keep fat and calories to a minimum and nutrition and flavor to the max, consider the following:

- Roast, broil, or grill meats and poultry, allowing the fat to drip away from the food as it cooks. You can buy a stovetop grill pan with a ridged bottom for this purpose.

- Poach chicken, seafood, or eggs in a nonfat or low-fat liquid, such as water, wine, juice, or low-fat broth. Poaching keeps food moist and flavorful without adding fat.

- Baking can be a healthy way to cook meat, poultry, and seafood without adding fat.

- Braising and stewing are slow-cooking methods that tenderize tough cuts of meat. Because the fat usually cooks out of meat or poultry, cook the dish a day ahead and chill it overnight. Chilling makes the fat rise to the top and harden, so you can remove it easily before reheating the dish.

- Steaming is a perfect way to cook seafood or vegetables without fat while retaining the food's natural flavor, vitamins, and minerals.

- Sautéing or stir-frying lets you cook meat or vegetables quickly over high heat with little or no fat. A nonstick finish on your skillet or wok comes in handy here.

- Microwave cooking is easy. It helps the food retain moisture and requires little or no added fat.

- Trim the fat from meat and remove the skin from poultry.

- Use water-packed canned fish and fruit.

Is your favorite recipe a little heavy in the calorie and fat department? Then trim it down by making the changes in the box on page 86.

fat-trimmers

INSTEAD OF USING	USE
Butter, lard, bacon or bacon fat, or chicken fat	Acceptable margarine or oil— margarine with no more than 2 grams of saturated fat per tablespoon or canola, olive, safflower, sunflower, or corn oil
Sour cream	Nonfat or light sour cream; nonfat or low-fat plain yogurt; puréed nonfat cottage cheese, thinned with a little fat-free milk or buttermilk
Whole milk	Fat-free milk
Whole-milk cheeses	Fat-free or low-fat cheeses
Whole eggs	2 egg whites for each whole egg; egg substitute
Heavy cream (1 cup)	1 cup fat-free evaporated milk; ½ cup nonfat or low-fat plain yogurt plus ½ cup nonfat cottage cheese
Cream cheese	Nonfat cream cheese, Neufchâtel cheese, or light cream cheese
Unsweetened baking chocolate (1-ounce square)	3 tablespoons unsweetened cocoa powder plus 1 tablespoon polyunsaturated oil or margarine

ORDERING À LA HEART

Sometimes eating out can torpedo your weight-loss efforts. We've developed some helpful hints about trimming fat from restaurant foods:

- When ordering food, be assertive and politely ask for what you want. Ask for margarine instead of butter, vegetables without butter, and dry toast.

- Ask to have gravies, sauces, and salad dressings served on the side, so you can control how much you eat.

- Ask how the food is prepared. For example, if the menu lists fried fish, ask whether the kitchen will broil yours instead. Many restaurants are happy to accommodate their customers.

- In Mexican food restaurants that serve complimentary fried tortilla chips, ask your waiter instead for soft corn tortillas to dip into the salsa. They have much less fat and fewer calories.

- Watch out for fast foods. Burgers and pizzas are loaded with fat and calories. Try submarine sandwiches with fresh ingredients, salads with a moderate amount of dressing, and stir-fried vegetables instead.

Also examine the descriptions of foods for clues about their fat and calorie content. See the box on page 88 for high-fat and low-fat clues.

de-coding the menu

HIGH-FAT CLUES	LOW-FAT CLUES
Au gratin, in cheese sauce, Parmesan	Au jus, in its own juice
Breaded and fried	Broiled with lemon juice or wine
Buttered, buttery, butter sauce	Baked
Creamed, creamy, in sauce	Fresh, garden fresh
Fried, deep fried, pan fried, french fried, batter fried, crispy	Grilled
Gravy, pan gravy	Lean
Hash	Poached
Hollandaise	Roasted
Pastry	Steamed
Pot pie	
Rich	
Sautéed	
Scalloped, escalloped	

THINK THIN

One final secret about food: You are what you think. When you're overeating, all you can think about is food. Not only do you consume it, it consumes you.

When you're not overeating, you think about lots of other things—fun activities, friends, parties, passions, hobbies, making a difference in the world, love, and meaning. Food is on the list, to be sure. But it's not at the top. It's sprinkled along like a spice, interweaving all the other priorities and joys of your life.

As a soon-to-be-healthier person, rethink your life and what's important to you. Then live it every day. What a difference!

5. JUST MOVE

Because it helps you burn stored fat, your best ally in the flab fight is exercise. Every brisk walk around the block, every pickup basketball game, or every dance step puts you closer to your healthiest and best-looking weight. As we pointed out earlier, when you burn more calories in activity than you take in from food, you lose weight.

The combination of eating less and exercising more is a powerful weight-loss tool. Here is the way to compute the average number of daily calories you need to maintain weight depending on your activity level:

- *To maintain your body weight:* Multiply the number of pounds you weigh now by 15. This represents the average number of calories used in one day if you're moderately active.

- *To maintain your body weight if you get very little exercise:* Multiply your weight by 13 instead of 15. Less-active people burn fewer calories.

With this information, you can balance your calorie intake and the number of calories you burn in physical activity to give yourself a small deficit every day. That is, if you need 1,500 calories a day to maintain your weight, eat 1,200 to 1,300 calories a day and walk or exercise more often. By eating 200 to 300 calories less and burning 200 to 300 more in exercise each day, you should achieve a weight loss that will be steady, sure, and *relatively* painless.

YOU DON'T HAVE TO BE A SUPERJOCK

In addition to cutting back on calories, adding physical activity will help you begin to lose weight at a steady clip. In fact, most people who've lost weight and kept it off for a year or more exercise for 45 to 60 minutes every day. Exercise speeds up your metabolism by increasing the amount of energy you expend in a day. Exercise helps your body burn calories more quickly, and if you're active shortly before a meal, the activity may help reduce your appetite.

When you start on a low-calorie diet, your metabolic rate tends to slow down. Your body is trying to burn calories more slowly because you're taking in fewer of them. Your body is saying, "Yikes! I'm starving. Better hold on to my reserves." Exercise helps minimize this slowdown by training your muscles to use fat to meet your energy needs. You'll burn calories more efficiently, which helps weight loss and reduces the breakdown of protein in the muscles.

Scientists have recently concluded that the "creeping obesity" seen in so many Americans—the tendency to gain a pound or two a year over several decades—is not related to age at all. Instead, evidence shows that this gradual weight gain is directly linked to the steady decline in physical activity and muscle mass that occurs as the average American enters middle age. In other words, if you never slowed down, you'd never gain weight. That's just one more reason why lifelong exercise is the way to go.

---

jill's story:
EXPERIMENTING WITH DIFFERENT EXERCISES

People who know Jill in her new slender life have trouble believing it, but all on her own, Jill lost 58 pounds. "I started noticing how out of breath I was and how my weight was affecting me physically. I decided that I needed to make a change, not only so I would look better, but so I would feel better too," said Jill, a 30-year-old music teacher.

When she was just out of college and in a new city with a new job, Jill decided to lose weight. She started educating herself about food, how it works, and what it does. She also started reading nutrition labels to find out the fat and calorie content of the foods she was eating. She started checking serving sizes. Now, rather than eating a hamburger and french fries for lunch, she chooses to eat a grilled chicken breast and salad.

Once she began to understand nutrition and follow her new way of eating, she started adding exercise to her program. "I opened my mind and started trying different exercises to find the one that worked for me," Jill said. "I tried walking, step aerobics, cycling at the gym, and racquet-ball." She even became a certified aerobics instructor and taught a few classes every week. This way, she had no excuse not to exercise; it was her job. Another way she stays active is by volunteering for events that encourage physical activity, such as the American Heart Walk.

By changing her eating habits and incorporating exercise into her life, she began to lose weight. "Once I saw that it worked, I tried doing a little more," Jill said. "I also began to notice that lean people have a different lifestyle than heavy people. They go to different restaurants and hang out at different places.

"I also continually reward myself for eating well and exercising," Jill said. "Rewarding myself has become a part of my life, just like eating healthier and exercising. If I follow my eating plan for a few days, I'll reward myself by spending a little extra money on new jeans that I can now fit into or buying a pair of shoes that I want but don't need."

Jill has also realized that changing her way of life has affected her overall well-being. "When I was heavier, I had no self-esteem and never went anywhere except to restaurants to eat," Jill said. "Now that I've lost weight, I am more outgoing, and people notice me. I also carry myself more confidently and am no longer afraid to go talk to a cute guy I see across the room."

If you're like most people who reach their goal weight, you'll want to make exercise a permanent part of your life. It not only helps keep the weight off but also offers dramatic health benefits that can protect you from the diseases that plague most Americans. Be sure to read our chapter on exercise, page 115. You'll see the powerful benefits of regular physical activity as well as the pure *fun* you can have. You'll even get excellent ideas on specific exercises to help you keep your new shape.

6. DRUM UP SUPPORT

Advice from the experts: Don't go it alone. Although rugged individualism is admirable, it can be highly overrated. When it comes to changing your life, everyone needs a good cheering section. This may take the form of supportive family, friends, and coworkers or a formal weight-loss program.

Think back to the hardest times in your life and the people who helped you: the coach who helped you make it through high school, the mentor who showed you how to handle office politics, the friend who lent an ear while you were going through a divorce. No matter what the outcome, supportive people encourage, comfort, and praise you. They help you put your failures into perspective. They help you stay focused on the goal. And they help you keep self-recrimination down and self-esteem up. Supportive people will lend emotional support and clear-thinking advice when you're tempted to binge, stop exercising, adopt fad diets, or anything else that will steer you wrong.

Best of all, a supportive friend can actually help you make a commitment to yourself. Together, you and your friend can sign a contract to see you through this process—no matter what. Use the following Commitment Agreement as a model. Draw up one that works for you. Get a support partner and enter into this agreement together. Support for changing your life is priceless, and it will see you through the rough times like nothing else.

COMMITMENT AGREEMENT

I, [*your name here*], agree that for as long as it takes, I will:

- Make losing weight a top priority, placing this need above the needs of others when necessary and appropriate.

- Maintain an enthusiastic, success-oriented attitude and avoid complaining, rejecting suggestions out of hand, and consciously or subconsciously seeking permission to backslide.

- Gather support for my weight-loss efforts at home, at work, and wherever else I need it. I will invite my support person to join me in activities designed to help my weight-loss efforts. (This could be exercise, cooking, or eating right.)

- Alter my eating plan and exercise plan to lose weight at a gradual but steady pace.

- Notice my emotions and deal with them in a way that will help me stay on target.

- Take responsibility for finding solutions to my weight-loss problems.

- Think positively and acknowledge my daily successes.

- Contact my support person, [*name of support person here*], at least once a week to report progress and share feelings.

I, [*name of support person here*], agree that for as long as it takes, I will:

- Support my friend's weight-loss efforts in every way possible, including maintaining a positive, accepting attitude and avoiding making judgments or criticizing.

- Participate in mutually agreed-upon activities, including eating right and exercising, modeling these behaviors for my friend.

- Help my friend to deal with emotional challenges and stressful situations, providing encouragement, praise, suggestions, and a listening ear when necessary.

- Help my friend think positively and acknowledge daily successes.

- Contact my friend at least once a week to offer interest, support, and encouragement.

Signed: _____
                                                    [*You*]

Date: _____

Signed: _____
                                        [*Support Person*]

Date: _____

7. HOW TO BACKSLIDE SUCCESSFULLY

How can you backslide? Let us count the ways: holidays, vacations, arguments, illness, stress, guilt, out-of-town visitors, gifts of food, celebrations, a death in the family, loss of a job, divorce, accident, major illness . . . and the list goes on.

At one time or another, you *will* backslide. That's just the way it goes. The important thing to remember about backsliding is that *it's just temporary*. As soon as the holiday is over, the visitors leave, you find another job, or the argument is resolved, go back to your new way of eating. Don't beat yourself up; just go back to eating like a healthy, slender person for life. You've already made the choice to do so. It's what you really want, so simply return.

FEND OFF EXTERNAL CUES

Experts tell us that people who are overweight generally react to external factors (the sight of food, the smell of freshly baked cookies) when deciding whether to eat. People of normal weight react more to internal factors, such as their own hunger. For that reason, controlling these cues helps you modify your eating behavior. For example:

- Make eating an activity in itself. Don't pair it with other activities such as watching television or reading.

- Establish an eating place, preferably at the table, and eat *only* there. Eliminate in-front-of-the-refrigerator munching.

- Keep food out of sight—in the pantry or refrigerator.

- Make a grocery list and stick to it.

- Plan for moments of weakness by stocking quick low-calorie munchables, such as cut-up carrots, cucumbers, radishes, green peppers, nonfat popcorn, pretzels, and low-fat crackers.

- Keep a list of projects you can do instead of eating to relieve tension. Then reach for the list instead of food.

- Don't let yourself get tired. It makes you want to eat as a pick-me-up. Get plenty of rest and sleep.

- Eat at least three regular, healthful meals a day. Keep all your meals about the same size. Add morning, afternoon, and evening snacks when you need them. Avoid getting too hungry—it's an invitation to backslide.

- Eat slowly. It takes 20 minutes for the food you eat to signal your brain that you're full. Eat what you now know is a normal meal. Then even if you don't feel full, put on the brakes. Wait the 20 minutes before eating more.

HOW TO BEAT BACKSLIDING

Amazingly, two-thirds of all backsliding occurs within 90 days of starting your new healthful way of eating. Events or situations usually trigger the backsliding. These high-risk situations are common to us all—they may just seem more difficult while you're trying to exchange your old overweight life for a new healthy-weight life. In general, high-risk situations fall into two categories: those happening within you and your environment and those happening between you and others.

You may suffer frustration, sadness, anger, worry, or boredom as a result of any number of difficult situations. The prospect of public speaking, trouble at work, a bounced check, or a car accident may send you scurrying to the pantry or the refrigerator. Illness or fatigue—what an excuse to drown your sorrows in ice cream! On the other hand, celebrating a birthday can also tempt you to indulge in ice cream. It doesn't matter whether it's the pain of being alone, the pleasure of being with friends, or the social pressure to indulge—each of us has emotional triggers that push us into old habits. For this reason, it's crucial that you learn to cope with painful emotions and acquire skills for resolving conflicts and dealing with peer pressures.

backsliding styles:
CHERYL'S, JERRY'S, AND DEBRA'S STORIES

When Cheryl's husband is in a bad mood or refuses to communicate with her, Cheryl becomes anxious and upset. To soothe these feelings, she cooks. Even when her weight-loss efforts are paying off, she cooks to overcome these unpleasant feelings—and, of course, she cooks fattening foods and eats what she cooks.

Jerry is great when he starts his eating plan. He joins a formal program, gets support, shows up at meetings, and starts losing two or three pounds a week. He is extremely enthusiastic and is eager to please his wife by fitting into his old swim trunks by summer. By the twelfth week, Jerry's enthusiasm has waned. This weight-loss effort is boring, the group is boring, and counting calories is boring, so he starts eating in the old way—and gaining weight.

Debra goes great guns on her diet. She's losing weight and dedicated to the process. Then one day she opens her pantry and finds a box of chocolates she thought she had thrown out. Immediately she begins to fantasize how the candy would taste. She decides to eat just one. Then one becomes two, three, seven, and finally the entire box.

We have three people and three different backsliding styles. Cheryl must realize that she backslides from *tension,* so she must find ways to deal with it other than cooking and eating. Jerry backslides from *boredom,* so he must launch into positive self-talk and stay motivated. Debra backslides from *visual stimulation,* so she must be careful to keep tempting food out of her home and avoid visually stimulating food scenarios such as looking at television commercials for food. No matter what, our backsliders must return to their new eating plans as soon as possible after backsliding.

---

8. WHAT'S EATING YOU?

When it comes to gaining weight, the key is not always what you're eating. It could be what's eating *you.* Painful emotions, such as depression, anxiety, anger, and loneliness, can contribute to overeating and bingeing. And irrational beliefs influence these emotions.

An emotion is actually a physical arousal that you can give a label, such as love, hate, joy, fear, or anger. Events or memories can trigger emotions. If an event has caused the emotion, you can get a handle on your reaction in several ways. You can:

Interpret the event so that you don't automatically get upset

Use self-talk to calm yourself and focus on taking action

Try deep breathing, progressive relaxation, meditation, exercise, or guided imagery

If a memory has caused the emotion, you can refuse to entertain it by immediately turning your thoughts elsewhere. Sometimes, despite your best efforts, you will find yourself feeling overwhelmed. When this happens, it's often from depression or anxiety, two core difficulties that you must examine and face.

COPING WITH DEPRESSION

Many overweight people suffer from depression. The signs include disturbed sleep, binge eating, extreme fatigue, agitation, or emotional flatness.

Depression is often triggered by real or imagined misfortunes, failures, defeats, or losses. It's normal to feel appropriately unhappy after one of these events, but if the depression doesn't lift after a reasonable amount of time—weeks or months, depending on the event's severity—you'll want to seek the help of a mental-health professional.

If you suspect you may be depressed, talk with your doctor or a mental-health professional. Any of these signs may mean depression: sleep problems, feeling overwhelmed, lack of energy or appetite, overeating, or lack of interest in sex or work.

If you are thinking about suicide, you need immediate professional help.

HIGH ANXIETY

Lisa gained 50 pounds shortly after her second marriage. Whenever she tried to lose weight, she developed severe attacks of anxiety and gave up. "As soon as I start losing weight, this huge fear I can't identify grips me," she explained. "My hands shake, I can't concentrate or even function. Only when I stop trying to lose weight does the fear go away."

In contrast to depression, which may be a response to *loss*, anxiety is a response to a *threat*. The threat may be real, imagined, exaggerated, or unknown. Anxiety shows up as tension and can include cold, clammy hands; shallow breathing; and tremors. The person with anxiety is often unable to concentrate and is withdrawn, restless, and preoccupied. If this preoccupation is intruded upon, the person becomes irritable. People with anxiety often have a sense of powerlessness or inability to cope. Their minds often race, repeatedly thinking the same catastrophic thoughts or painful images. In severe cases, people feel panicky, faint, or dizzy or have chest pains, nausea, diarrhea, or headaches.

Some anxiety is natural. You're facing a stressful event, so the anxiety is your signal to prepare yourself to cope with it effectively. If you're facing a past stressful event—something from your childhood, perhaps—anxiety is your signal to resolve this issue. If anxiety interferes with your ability to function effectively day to day or if you have debilitating symptoms, you need to get help from a mental-health professional.

WHAT CAN YOU DO?

We have good news. You can take steps to combat mild depression and mild anxiety, gaining perspective on your life and reducing their hold on you. The following self-help ideas are tried and true—so try them on for size. Do talk with your doctor or a mental-health professional if you think you have serious problems with depression or anxiety.

Change illogical thought patterns

Carefully examine the basis of your depression or the threat that has you feeling anxious. Is your depression caused by the loss of a person or a job? If you don't know why you're depressed, talk with a mental-health professional. Is your threat real, imagined, exaggerated, or unknown? Too often, your own thoughts or imagination may bring on depression or anxiety.

Learn to relax

Try deep breathing, meditation, guided imagery, yoga, or any activity that will help you relax deeply. You'll know you've relaxed because you'll have less muscle tension, slower breathing, slower heart rate, and a more peaceful mind.

Progressive deep-muscle relaxation also works. This involves sitting or lying comfortably and tensing each part of your body, holding the tension for a few seconds, then letting go of the tension. Continue tensing and relaxing your face, neck, arms, hands, shoulders, chest, abdomen, buttocks, legs, and feet. Finally, tense and relax the whole body at once, noticing how different your body feels during each stage of the exercise. When you've completed the exercise, let yourself enjoy the feeling of total relaxation for a few minutes before getting up.

Clear your mind

Some call it meditation. Others call it a mental break. In either case, clearing your mind for 20 minutes each day does wonders for your mental health. Simply sit comfortably in relaxed clothing. Remove your glasses. Breathe deeply for a minute or two.

Focus on your breath as it goes out. You may want to focus only on the breath, with no other thoughts. Perhaps you'd rather concentrate on a single thought: "Love" or "Calm" or "Let go." Some people like to concentrate on an image such as a beach or a meadow. If other thoughts intrude, just label them "thinking" and gently let them go, returning to the outbreath, the word, or the image you have chosen. If you do this for 10 to 20 minutes a day, you'll feel refreshed, energetic, and ready for life. It also has an overall calming effect and helps you handle day-to-day pressures with greater composure and serenity.

Exercise regularly

We've said it before, and we'll say it again: Exercise is amazing. It promotes good health, calmness, and relaxation. Please read our chapter on exercise, page 115. It will give you the lowdown on how to pick yourself up.

---

keiko's story:
WHAT DEPRESSION CAN DO

"I got married and came to this country to live," said Keiko, who left her family, friends, and job in Japan. She knew no one but her husband in the United States. "In six months I ballooned from 102 pounds to 138 pounds. I was scared about what was happening to me," she recalled. She realized that she was lonely and depressed and that she had turned to food for comfort.

She started watching her portion sizes. She learned to cut down on fat and sugar in cooking and to add herbs and spices for flavor. She ate lots of raw vegetables to help fill her stomach.

"At first, I was weighing myself every week, but I didn't see a lot of progress. It was making me crazy," she said. She stopped weighing. She started walking the dog. It took her five years, but she got back to 102 pounds. That was 10 years ago. When she gets up to 107 pounds, she starts eating less and walking more.

"It still takes willpower," she said. She practices by keeping a bowl of candy on her desk and *not eating it!* "When I'm going out to eat or to a party with friends, I eat a piece of fruit or drink vegetable juice before I go. I know I'll eat party food, but I'll eat less if I'm not ravenous when I get there." If she eats a candy bar in the afternoon, she makes up for it at dinner by having fruit instead of dessert.

"It's a lifetime struggle, but it's well worth staying in control," she said.

---

9. CAN WE TALK?

One of the most powerful weight-loss secrets is the art of *positive self-talk*. The plain truth is that people actually do what they tell themselves to do. For example, Janna wanted to lose the extra 40 pounds she'd been carrying since she had her baby. Losing that much weight seemed like an uphill battle to her. She'd tell herself things like:

- "I'll never be able to lose 40 pounds."

- "I wish I could eat like Bill and not gain weight."

- "Everyone at that table is having a big, luscious dessert. I think I'll have one too."

- "I don't have time to lose weight now."

- "I ate the whole bag of cookies. I'll never be able to pull this off."

This negative self-talk pulled her down. It sounded so true that she'd give in to it and literally do what she "talked herself into."

accentuate the positive—eliminate the negative

NEGATIVE SELF-TALK	POSITIVE SELF-TALK
"I'll never be able to lose 40 pounds."	"You don't have to lose 40 pounds all at once; your blood pressure will be better if you lose even 10. Remember that your goal is to be healthier. Just take it one day at a time."
"I wish I could eat like Bill and not gain weight."	"You have your own body and genes. Life is not always fair, but you owe it to yourself to keep your body as healthy as possible."

NEGATIVE SELF-TALK	POSITIVE SELF-TALK
"Everyone at that table is having a big, luscious dessert. I think I'll have one too."	"You need to pay your bill and leave. You know that losing weight is more important to you than tasting a rich dessert."
"I don't have time to lose weight now."	"You will always be busy. Sit down with your calendar and choose a time to start losing weight. Then you'll just have to fit it in around your activities."
"I ate the whole bag of cookies. I'll never be able to pull this off."	"You just had a momentary lapse. You can pick yourself up and make a fresh start."

From that day forward, Janna vowed to turn all negative self-talk into positive self-talk. It was difficult at first, but soon became second nature. In time, she "talked" herself into a new, smaller dress size.

Good losers have actually used self-talk to their advantage—sometimes with dramatic results. Try these on for size:

Create your own self-fulfilling prophecy

Patti lost 35 pounds in a formal weight-loss program. "The greatest thing I learned from the program was to say, 'I can.' I can do anything I set my mind to do. And I did!"

Avoid temptation

Jerry was constantly tempted by ice cream. When confronted by the lure of a sundae, he now tells himself, "I no longer have to shop in a big-men's store. I lost weight and look good!" Soon the desire for the ice cream passes.

Build yourself up

When you're overweight, it's easy to put yourself down. Positive self-talk can pick you up again. Christine used to say, "Nobody likes me because I'm fat." Now she says, "Everyone, including me, is special and unique. I like who I am."

Sidestep food cravings

Sometimes you'll think of a food and then crave it. You can't stop thinking about it until you have it. Kayla, who permanently lost weight 11 years ago, says when tempted, "Nothing tastes as good as thin feels!" She also asks herself, "Which means more—eating this or becoming healthy and slender?" No contest!

Steer clear of "poor me"

It's easy to feel deprived when you're losing weight. The illusion is that everyone—except you—can eat whatever he or she wants. Karen, who lost 63 pounds, uses positive self-talk to avoid that "poor me" feeling about chocolate, a food that's almost impossible for her to eat in small quantities. "I tell myself that this is one thing I can't have," said Karen. "Lactose intolerant people can't have milk, and I can't have chocolate. It's no big deal."

10. SLENDER: NOT JUST A WORD, BUT A LIFESTYLE

Permanently slender people don't go on or off "diets." That's because they live a lifestyle that naturally promotes healthful eating and a healthy weight. To them, eating right, getting regular exercise, engaging in positive self-talk, and personal effectiveness and self-determination are just part of everyday life.

---

betty's story:
SHE'LL NEVER GO BACK

About the time of Betty's divorce, she took stock of her life. As part of her inventory, she weighed herself. "I was shocked—I weighed 172 pounds. I had no idea because I never weighed myself. I didn't want to know," she said.

Betty joined a weight-loss program at work. She completely changed her eating habits, and she started walking twice a day. Her dogs made the walking part easy.

Over the next year and a half, she lost 42 pounds. That was 12 years ago. Today she still eats the same menu she devised for herself then. Weekdays she has cereal, fruit, fat-free milk, and juice for breakfast. For lunch she has a big salad that she takes from home. For dinner she has a chicken breast, lean meat, or fish; one or two vegetables, usually including broccoli; and a baked potato, rice, or pasta. Then she splurges a little on the weekend. She also allows herself a variety of foods when she travels—two or three times a year. Pleased that she has the energy to enjoy new places and new sights, she treats herself to a trip to Europe every other year.

At home, it doesn't matter to her that she has a routine menu. "This is the menu I lost weight on, and I don't want to mess with it. I might start gaining again," she says. Since she cooks for one, having a basic pattern to follow every week makes meal planning and shopping very easy.

She says she has kept the weight off through sheer determination. "If I make up my mind to do something, that's it. I do it."

———————————————————————

Now that you have the tools, all you need is commitment to live a healthful lifestyle in a slender body. Make a commitment to yourself and to the process. You can do it.

getting
OFF YOUR
ROCKER

how to dump your couch-potato
lifestyle and really start living

> "WE MUST BECOME
>   THE CHANGE WE WANT TO SEE."
>   — MAHATMA GANDHI

"THIS YEAR," YOU SAY, "I'M GOING TO GET MORE EXERCISE."

So right away you find the nearest health club. The first week, you take the place by storm: 45 minutes on the treadmill and 30 minutes of weight training every day. The second week, you skip a day. By the fourth week, you're going every other day. In a couple of months, that drops to once or twice a week, and finally you quit altogether. Sound familiar?

This is not too surprising. Why? Because this scenario is *not* the way to make regular physical activity part of your everyday life. In fact, it's a prescription for failure.

"No Pain, No Gain" Is a Pain

The main reason you don't stick with this exercise program is that it's simply *not fun for you*. People who make physical activity a regular part of their lives— we call them "good movers"—succeed because they choose an activity they *really like*. They start slowly, then gradually increase the time and intensity. This approach is gentle but steady. Ultimately, you get all the gain without a lot of pain.

For example, Maria's hobby is gardening. She loves flowers and flower arranging. Although lifting and digging in her garden helped Maria build strength, it didn't do much for her cardiovascular system. She began walking regularly through the city parks and the arboretum. At first, she walked slowly, looking at all the plants and flowers, but she built up to a brisk walk. She was having so much fun that she hardly noticed she was exercising 30 to 60 minutes a day four or five days a week!

Her neighbor Sean had been on his high school swim team and loved it. However, after 20 years of beer, high-fat snacks, and television watching from his easy chair, Sean was out of shape. Remembering his high school days, he joined the YMCA and started swimming laps in its Olympic-size pool. After several months, he was regularly swimming for an hour or more at least three days a week—and having a great time.

"Great for them," you say, "but my hobby is stamp collecting." Okay, so your interests don't exactly promote physical activity. No problem. You simply build some kind of activity into your life. Choose something that will give you a fun break from your sedentary hobbies. Walk in your neighborhood and speak to your neighbors. Enjoy the trees, flowers, birds, and squirrels or the shops, office buildings, and parks. Take your children or grandchildren to the park—and keep up with them!

Tony's hobby is collecting baseball memorabilia, a hobby that is mostly sedentary. To get some exercise, Tony went to his nearest recreation center and signed up to play in a beginner's basketball league. The coach was encouraging, and the games were a blast. In a few months Tony was good enough for the intermediate league. Between weekly practices and games, he gets from four to six hours of strong cardiovascular workout every week—and he has such a good time that he doesn't even think of it as exercise.

If you've been sedentary for a long time, the phrase "physical activity" may conjure up memories of gym classes with boring push-ups or softball games in which you couldn't catch or hit the ball. You may remember always being the last person picked to be on a team. You may not have had the skills or training you needed or the support of the coach to enjoy participating in these activities. Also, many of us have the idea that only successful athletes enjoy physical activity.

Fortunately, experts now recognize that regardless of your age—from 2 to 92—you can develop a lifelong pattern for movement if you try a wide variety of activities. Physical education teachers now work at introducing students to activities they can do individually, without having lots of other people to make up a team. Many students learn to enjoy running, swimming, cycling, tennis, dancing, and other kinds of exercise that interest them.

Many of us have a doctor in the background prescribing more exercise. If this is not true for you, it's always a good idea to get your doctor's okay before adding regular physical activity—particularly if you've been totally sedentary or if the activity is especially vigorous.

THREE WAYS TO RECOGNIZE A GOOD MOVER

GOOD MOVERS TRY NEW PURSUITS

Good movers are pleasure seekers. They search out new and different activities that they enjoy. Never tried fencing? Give it a whirl. Soccer, badminton, hiking, folk dancing, sailing, downhill skiing—the list is endless. Having options makes it less likely that you'll abandon exercise after an illness or vacation. And it makes life more interesting!

GOOD MOVERS MAKE IT DIFFICULT NOT TO EXERCISE

These creative people arrange their lives to accommodate exercise. They carry workout clothing and shoes in their car or keep a pair of walking shoes at work. They post activity notices on their refrigerator. They put sports equipment out in plain sight to remind themselves to play. Instead of avoiding unnecessary movement ("While you're up, would you get me a beer?") they *embrace* unnecessary movement ("I'll go" or "Let me get it").

GOOD MOVERS EXERCISE TO FEEL BETTER

Good movers have discovered that exercise should make you feel better. Choose activities that make you feel as good when you finish as when you started—maybe better! If they don't, make them less intense or try something different.

The Pleasure Principle: Find an Activity That's "Fun and Games"

You can put pep in your step—and fun in your life—by finding activities that perk up your attitude as well as your body. Here are some engaging activities that can lure even the most dedicated sofa spud:

Aerobic dancing	Cross-country skiing
Bicycling	Swimming
Hiking	Rowing
Jumping rope	Running
In-line or ice skating	Using a treadmill
Jogging	Skateboarding
Stair climbing	Snowboarding
Walking	

If you're sports-oriented, here are some activities to check out:

Tennis	Basketball
Squash	Volleyball
Soccer	Lacrosse
Badminton	Gymnastics
Ice hockey	Downhill skiing
Racquetball	

You may choose less-vigorous activities, but do them longer and more often than you would the more-vigorous types. The good news is that you can still get most of the same health benefits as long as you do them often enough (see "Good News for Nonjocks," page 123). These less-vigorous activities or sports may catch your imagination:

Fencing	Diving
Softball	Archery
Bowling	Golf
Square dancing	Horseback riding
Scuba diving	Sailing
Table tennis	Surfing
Tai chi	Windsurfing
Yard work	Yoga

---

spencer's story:
FITTING IN FITNESS AT THE WORKPLACE

"I didn't get much activity in my job," said Spencer, a network administrator. "I spent most of my days in front of the computer and most of my evenings in front of the television."

Spencer, who was about 30 pounds overweight, had been unhappy with the way he looked and finally decided to do something about it. "I knew that I wouldn't stick to a formal exercise program, so I started thinking of ways I could just become more active in my everyday life," he said.

He started by taking the stairs at work. "Anytime I wanted a drink or made a photocopy, I would take the stairs to a different floor. That made me get up out of my chair and get a little exercise," said Spencer.

After a few weeks, he began taking 15 minutes during his lunch break to walk around the office building. "By taking the stairs and walking during lunch, I was getting almost 30 minutes of exercise each day," said Spencer. "I've found that it's an easy exercise program to fit into my day, and that's just what I needed. I've also lost some weight and have been able to keep it off."

Good News for Nonjocks

Everyone knows you have to be a marathon runner to get the health benefits of exercise, right? Wrong! The latest research shows that people who are moderately active on a regular basis can still reap many of the health benefits enjoyed by their more vigorous buddies (see chart on pages 124 and 125).

what it takes to reap health benefits

Washing and waxing a car for 45 to 60 minutes

Washing windows or mopping floors for 45 to 60 minutes

Playing volleyball for 45 minutes

Playing touch football for 30 to 45 minutes

Gardening for 30 to 45 minutes

Wheeling yourself in a wheelchair for 30 to 45 minutes

Walking 1¾ miles in 35 minutes (20 minutes per mile)

Shooting baskets for 30 minutes

Bicycling 5 miles in 30 minutes

Dancing fast (social dancing) for 30 minutes

Pushing a baby in a stroller 1½ miles in 30 minutes (20 minutes per mile)

Raking leaves for 30 minutes

Less Vigorous, More Time

Walking 2 miles in 30 minutes
(15 minutes per mile)

Doing water aerobics for
30 minutes

Swimming laps for 20 minutes

Playing wheelchair basketball
for 20 minutes

Playing basketball for 15 to
20 minutes

Bicycling 4 miles in 15 minutes
(3¾ minutes per mile)

Jumping rope for 15 minutes

Running 1½ miles in 15 minutes
(10 minutes per mile)

More Vigorous,
Less Time

Research shows that just being *more active*—in any way—can help you look and feel better and reduce your risk of heart disease. For example, you'll be more active if you take the stairs instead of the elevator, walk into the bank instead of using the drive-up window, park as far from the mall entrance as you can, take your own groceries to the car and load them in, and walk to the airport gate instead of taking a shuttle or a moving sidewalk.

Best of all, the studies say you don't have to do all

your physical activity at one time. Instead of walking 30 minutes once a day, for example, you can split the walk into three 10-minute segments. If you can manage to work in an *accumulated* total of 30 minutes or more of moderate activity each day, you can get most of the health benefits of a more vigorous exercise program.

You have a *choice:* You can get the health benefits of exercise by doing longer sessions of moderately intense activity (walking 1¾ miles in 35 minutes) or shorter sessions of more vigorous activities (running 1½ miles in 15 minutes).

Prod Your Bod

The trick to getting all the health benefits of physical activity is to make sure you're doing it vigorously enough. The easiest way to measure your overall pace is to use the Effort Scale below. The scale goes from 0 to 9: a 0-level effort means you're not moving; a 9-level effort means you're moving as hard as you can—it's total exhaustion.

A healthy, brisk walking or exercise pace will usually put you at an effort level of 3 to 5. You feel it in your body, as if you're hurrying to catch a bus. For example, at level 3, you should feel as if:

- You're breathing faster than when you aren't exercising.

- You can talk in short sentences but can't sing.

- The exercise is comfortably hard.

If you exercise at this pace—or a little stronger—you'll be challenging yourself enough to get the health benefits you want. As you progress, you'll find yourself wanting to step up the pace. You'll want to work up to level 5 or 6 to get more benefit.

THE EFFORT SCALE

0	Nothing at all
1	Very light—GETTING OFF THE COUCH
2	Light
3	Moderate/brisk—BEGINNING TO ENJOY ACTIVITY
4	Somewhat hard
5	Hard—GETTING SERIOUS
6	Very hard
7	Very, very hard
8	Extremely hard
9	Maximum effort—YOU MUST BE CRAZY!

Your Target Heart Rate

To check on whether you're working hard enough in your exercise, the Effort Scale works well, especially in the beginning. If you want to get the *most* benefit for your heart and lungs out of any physical activity, however, you need to exercise at a level strenuous enough to raise your heart rate to your "target zone." Your *tar-*

get heart rate is 50 to 75 percent of your *maximum* heart rate, which is the fastest your heart can beat.

To find out whether you're exercising within your target heart rate zone, count the number of pulse beats at your wrist or neck for 10 seconds. Multiply by 6 to get the number of beats per minute. This number should be within your target heart rate zone. If it's too high, you're exercising too hard, and you should slow down. If it's too low, exercise a little harder.

To find your target zone, just look at the following chart.

TARGET HEART RATE*

Find your age or the age closest to yours, then read across the line. You'll see your average maximum heart rate (100%) and your target heart rate zone (50% to 75% of maximum).

AGE	AVG. MAX. HEART RATE	TARGET HEART RATE ZONE 50% TO 75% OF MAX.
20	200	100 to 150 beats per minute
25	195	98 to 146 beats per minute
30	190	95 to 142 beats per minute
35	185	93 to 138 beats per minute
40	180	90 to 135 beats per minute
45	175	88 to 131 beats per minute
50	170	85 to 127 beats per minute
55	165	83 to 123 beats per minute

AGE	AVG. MAX. HEART RATE	TARGET HEART RATE ZONE 50% TO 75% OF MAX.
60	160	80 to 120 beats per minute
65	155	78 to 116 beats per minute
70	150	75 to 113 beats per minute

NOTE: A few high-blood-pressure medicines lower the maximum heart rate and, thus, the target-zone rate. If you are taking a high-blood-pressure medication, ask your doctor what your target heart rate should be.

* *These figures are averages and should be used as general guidelines.*

When you first start exercising, aim for the lower end of your target zone: 50 percent of your maximum heart rate. As you get stronger and more active, build up to the higher end (75 percent of maximum). Some medications make it difficult for you to reach your target zone. If it's too hard for you to exercise at 50 to 75 percent, find a pace that's comfortable for you. In time, you may feel that you can slowly increase the intensity to reach your target zone. Always listen to your body, and don't try to do the impossible!

WARM-UPS AND COOL-DOWNS

If you plan to exercise vigorously, you'll want to start your session with a short warm-up. This may help keep you from getting hurt. All you have to do is walk slowly or jog for about five minutes, until your muscles are warmed up. Then stretch for a few moments to make sure your arms and legs are flexible and ready.

A cool-down is a warm-up in reverse. After your activity, make yourself slow down gradually, then walk slowly or jog for five minutes before stopping. This keeps the blood from pooling in your legs and allows your body to gradually return to normal.

Does Your Workout Measure Up?

HEALTH BENEFITS

Okay. All you need to do is accumulate *30 minutes of moderate physical activity on most days.* You can walk for 10 minutes before work, 10 minutes at lunchtime, and 10 minutes after work, and you're there. Or you can enlist your spouse or a friend and walk for 30 minutes every evening. Either way, you'll get your health benefits.

WEIGHT LOSS

This is a little tougher. Diet is important here. If you take in 200 to 300 calories less and burn 200 to 300 more in exercise every day, you should achieve a healthy, steady weight loss.

Take a look at the chart on page 131. You can see how many calories you burn during 30 minutes of various physical activities. Also remember that little bits of activity during the day push up the total calories spent.

GETTING FIT

For cardiovascular fitness, you'll want to do *30 to 45 minutes of vigorous physical activity 3 or 4 days a week*. That will give your heart and lungs the serious, sustained workout necessary to reach peak cardiovascular health.

CALORIES BURNED IN A 30-MINUTE WORKOUT

ACTIVITY	BODY WEIGHT (LB.)		
	100	150	200
Walking (2.0 mph or 30 min./mile)	84	120	156
Walking (3.0 mph or 20 min./mile)	112	160	208
Walking (4.5 mph)	154	220	286
Jogging (5.5 mph)	259	370	481
Running (6.0 mph or 10 min./mile)	448	640	832
Swimming (25 yds./min.)	97	138	179
Swimming (50 yd./min.)	175	250	325
Bicycling (6.0 mph or 10 min./mile)	84	120	156
Bicycling (12.0 mph or 5 min./mile)	144	205	267

NOTE: The more you weigh, the more calories you burn during physical activity, since a heavier body expends more energy.

What *Is* Fitness?

Fitness is a condition, not a program. It is having the energy to do all you want to do in life—and more. Fitness is what happens when you decide to include regular physical activity in your everyday life. When exercise becomes as much a part of your life as grooming or working, you will become fit.

True fitness has four basic parts:

1. *Aerobic fitness.* The ability of your heart and lungs to deliver enough oxygen to your muscles to produce the energy you need. Activities that promote aerobic fitness give your heart and lungs a workout. They include walking, jogging, running, bicycling, swimming, cross-country skiing, and stair climbing.

2. *Muscular fitness.* The strength and endurance of your muscles. Muscular fitness is critical to most daily tasks: carrying groceries, lifting a child, pushing a lawnmower. To get your muscles fit, you'll need activities that will help you improve the major muscles in both your upper and lower body. Weight lifting is an example.

3. *Flexibility.* The ability to bend your joints and stretch your muscles in a full range of motion. If you're not flexible, you can injure yourself easily, and your ability to move quickly and easily is limited. If you fall, you're more likely to hurt

yourself. Regular stretching exercises and yoga help loosen the major joints in your body.

4. *Body composition.* The amount of fat on your body compared to the amount of muscle and bone. In short, how much of your total weight is fat? Too much or too little fat can cause health problems that sidetrack your overall fitness.

HOW CAN I GET FIT?

You probably know a few fitness fanatics and avoid them like the plague. Don't worry. Becoming fit is not like going to Marine Corps boot camp. It's more like deciding to have fun. All it takes is four simple steps:

1. Find out if you're ready.
2. Create a *fun* plan to get fit—and stay with it.
3. Track your progress.
4. Decide to love your physical activity—choose to make it a regular part of your life.

ARE YOU READY TO GET FIT?

The first test is the most important—and that's testing your sincere desire and readiness to add regular physical activity to your life. If you haven't already done it, turn to page 6 and take our Stages of Change Test.

If you find you're not ready, explore some of the options suggested below the test. When you can uncover the reasons why changing your life for the better feels difficult, you'll be better able to work on those. Don't try to increase physical activity until you feel ready; you may be setting yourself up to fail. Instead, give yourself every advantage to succeed. If you're not ready to change your activity level, see if you might be ready to change your eating habits or give up smoking. Start with whatever feels most doable.

On the other hand, if the test shows you *are* ready to tackle physical activity, let's begin now! First, make sure you're physically ready too. Complete this quick Physical Activity Readiness Checklist:

Physical Activity Readiness Checklist
Mark the items that apply to you.

___Your doctor said you have a heart condition and recommended only medically supervised physical activity.

___During or right after you exercise, you frequently have pains or pressure in the left or midchest area, left side of the neck, or left shoulder or arm.

___You have developed chest pain within the last month.

___You tend to lose consciousness or fall over due to dizziness.

___You feel extremely breathless after mild exertion.

___Your doctor recommended you take medicine for your blood pressure or a heart condition.

___Your doctor said you have bone or joint problems that could be made worse by the proposed physical activity.

___You have a medical condition or other physical reason not mentioned here that might need special attention in an exercise program (such as insulin-dependent diabetes).

___You are a man over age 40 or a woman over age 50, have not been physically active, and plan a relatively vigorous exercise program.

If you checked even one of the items on the readiness list, you need to talk with your doctor before beginning any exercise program. If you develop any of the symptoms described above, see your doctor.

Walking:
The No-Sweat Workout

If you want to change your life and get fit, find a moderate or vigorous activity that's fun for you, and *start slowly.* Because walking is such a popular choice in the United States, we'll start with a simple walking plan. You can use this plan as a model for any activity you choose. The key is to go slowly and gradually increase your activity.

darren's story:
GRADUAL PROGRESS IS BEST

After hip surgery, Darren found it difficult to resume his active lifestyle. "I had always been an avid runner and physically active," he said. "But after my surgery, running was quite painful. Reluctantly, I began walking for exercise. I had always assumed walking wasn't challenging, even though I had never really tried walking vigorously for exercise."

He began walking 15 minutes each day for about two weeks. Then he started increasing the amount of time he walked, bumping it up a little every other week. Gradually, he walked his way up to 30 minutes a day. "I was surprised at how much walking helped me and how much I enjoyed it," Darren said. "I began regaining the strength in my legs and building up my stamina. It was a long road to recovery, but that was what worked best for me."

HOW TO WALK ALL OVER HEART DISEASE

When it comes to improving your life, your health, and your fitness level, you can hardly beat walking. In fact, it's probably the best all-around exercise. Walking is inexpensive, easy, and convenient. It's low-impact, yet it gives your heart and lungs a real workout—which makes it great for promoting aerobic fitness. Because walking is a weight-bearing exercise, it helps prevent bone loss. Carrying hand weights while walking can also help. It offers your upper body more resistance, so you can build muscle tone at the same time. If you stretch thoroughly before each walking session, you can improve your overall flexibility. Walking itself will help you keep your weight normal and regulate your body composition.

Whether you want to get healthy, lose weight, or get fit, the following easy walking plan is designed to get you there—gradually and painlessly. It starts with walking 15 minutes a day. You probably do that already without thinking about it. Now you'll do it deliberately.

THE AMERICAN HEART ASSOCIATION'S NO-SWEAT WALKING PLAN

SCHEDULE	TOTAL WALKING TIME	HOW OFTEN EACH WEEK
Week 1	15 minutes	3 or 4 days
Week 2	20 minutes	3 or 4 days
Week 3	20 minutes	4 or 5 days
Week 4	25 minutes	4 or 5 days
Week 5	30 minutes	4 or 5 days
Week 6	30 minutes	4 to 6 days
Ongoing	Increase to 45 minutes or more	4 to 6 days

You can start by walking the dog every evening, walking the circumference of your office building before work, finding a coworker and walking before lunch—anything that keeps you moving just 15 minutes every day. Each week you'll add five minutes to that daily total. Five minutes is nothing—you can get that by walking during your coffee break.

Just stick with the plan, and you'll be amazed at how quickly you get used to being more active. After a while, you'll feel so good you won't want to miss a single day of being active. If you do miss a day, don't sweat it. Get right back in the habit the next day. All gain, no pain.

---

yolanda's story:
FRIENDS MAKE A DIFFERENCE

"I had never been physically active and didn't want to be," said Yolanda, a 40-year-old producer. "After getting out of breath from everyday activities such as walking up stairs or carrying in groceries from my car, I decided it was time for a change."

As a mother of four, Yolanda didn't have much spare time in her life. "After carpooling, getting dinner on the table, and helping with homework, I was too exhausted in the evenings to even think of exercise," she said. "So I decided to start early in the morning while I had the time and energy." She began to get up a little earlier than usual and walk for about 15 minutes in the morning. "I mentioned to my neighbor what I was doing, and she decided to start walking with me," said Yolanda. "We soon worked our way up to walking thirty minutes each morning."

She soon noticed that some things were easier to do. "I no longer had to rest after walking up a flight of stairs," said Yolanda. "I was also able to keep up with my two-year-old much more easily than before."

Eventually, a few more neighbors joined in on walking. "Now there's a big group," said Yolanda. "It's made exercise a lot more fun for all of us. It's also made us responsible to someone other than ourselves for getting our exercise—no excuses allowed."

The great thing about walking is that you don't really need special clothing or shoes. You can wear just about anything that feels comfortable. If you want to make walking a permanent part of your life, however, it's a good idea to make your walks as comfortable as possible.

KEEP IT LOOSE AND LIGHT

Choose a wardrobe that's loose-fitting and light-weight. During summer, you may want to wear light-colored clothing to reflect the sun's rays, wear sunglasses, and use a waterproof sunscreen of at least SPF 15. Cotton clothing works best to help keep you cool because it absorbs perspiration. As the weather cools, add layers.

THE RIGHT SHOES

For each mile you walk, your feet hit the ground between 1,500 and 2,000 times. That's why athletic shoes are so popular. You'll find special shoes for walking, running, aerobic dance, cross training, and basketball. Walking shoes weigh about the same as running shoes, but they're usually lighter than the other three types. Americans buy more walking shoes than any other type of athletic shoe—more than 46 million pairs per year!

Walking shoes are so popular because their design allows for an easy heel-to-toe rocking motion. They have special cushioning that absorbs shock throughout the sole, especially in the heel. Walking shoes should be replaced every 500 to 600 miles (that's once a year if you walk 9 to 12 miles a week) or if:

- The tread pattern is worn smooth.

- The tread becomes overly worn, either on the inside or outside at the heel.

- The shoes don't feel as cushiony as when you first bought them.

- You start to develop pains in your hips, knees, or shins, and you haven't had an injury or changed your walking routine.

BUYING WALKING SHOES

When shopping for walking shoes, keep these tips in mind. They can help you get the comfort, style, and support you need.

- If you need special help and advice, visit an athletic footwear specialty store.

- Shop late in the day, when your feet are at their largest.

- If you have some old athletic shoes, bring them along when you shop. They will help the salesperson analyze your gait and the places of most wear. Then you can buy new shoes that match your gait.

- When trying on shoes, wear the socks you'll exercise in.

- Make sure the front of the shoe is wide enough so that your toes can spread easily.

- Press your thumb down at the tip of your longest toe to make sure the toe is about the width of a thumbnail from the end of the shoe.

- After lacing, make sure that the lace holes on either side of the shoe are at least one inch apart. If they're too close, you won't have enough room for adjustment. If they're more than a couple of inches apart, the shoes may be too tight.

- Stand on your tiptoes to make sure that your heel doesn't come out of the shoe.

- Walk briskly around the store to check for comfort and cushioning. Walk on a hard surface, if possible. Make sure that the shoe bends easily under the ball of your foot, there's no tightness or rubbing, and the shoe's arch support matches up with your foot's arch.

- Consider buying mesh or leather walking shoes; they let your feet breathe.

SOCK IT TO ME

For walking comfort and blister prevention, choose socks that fit without bunching. Be sure not to get them too small—they'll put too much pressure on the end of your toes. Acrylic socks are a good choice because they'll wick the sweat away from the surface of your skin. Cotton socks will hold the moisture at your feet and bunch when wet. The thickness really doesn't matter. Just be sure to try on shoes with the socks you'll be wearing; otherwise, the shoes may fit too loosely or too tightly.

YOUR WATER BOTTLE RUNNETH OVER

Anytime you're active, you'll want to drink plenty of water. That's because each time you breathe out, you lose moisture from your lungs. When you're walking briskly, your breathing rate increases—along with the moisture loss.

You also lose water through perspiration. That's how your body cools itself—as the sweat on your skin evaporates, it cools your skin's surface. Because the moisture evaporates so rapidly, you may not even notice that you're sweating. You're still losing fluid, so always drink plenty of water—whether you think you're sweating or not. Here are some hydration tips:

- Drink water, not caffeinated or alcoholic beverages. Caffeine and alcohol actually cause your body to lose water.

- Drink 6 to 8 ounces of water right before and right after your physical activity.

- Experiment. If you're going for a long or fast walk in hot, humid weather, weigh yourself before and after you walk. The difference is due to water loss. You need to replace the lost water by drinking two cups of water for every pound lost.

- Water is all you really need. If you plan to be active for an hour or longer, you may want to have some fruit juice to replace potassium; try orange or cranberry juice mixed with an equal amount of water. Some people may prefer to use a sports drink.

- If you're going for a long walk, hike, or cross-country skiing trek, make sure you carry water with you. Most backpacks hold a water bottle, or you can buy a special belt with a similar holder. Be careful not to get dehydrated, especially on days when the temperature is 65°F or higher.

- Don't depend on thirst to tell you when to drink. You need it long before your body offers signals. If possible, drink water at 15- to 20-minute intervals during moderate or vigorous physical activity lasting an hour or more.

KEEP AN EYE ON THE WEATHER

When you're active every day, year-round, you'll run into all kinds of weather. These tips will show you the ropes on how to handle winter, summer, and rainy-weather woes.

Cold weather

- Warm up and stretch before going outdoors.

- Pay careful attention to the windchill factor and dress accordingly.

- In extreme cold or when the windchill is high, wear a hat, gloves, and thick socks. Wrap a scarf around your head, neck, and face.

- Wear sunglasses and sunscreen on bright sunny days.

- Keep your head covered, especially when the temperature is in the 30s or below.

- Dress in layers. Wearing too much is better than not wearing enough.

- Wear a windbreaker with a front zipper for the outer layer.

- Remove or open outer layers before sweating makes the under layers wet.

- If you get chilled, put a layer back on.

- If your clothing becomes wet for any reason, go indoors and change as soon as possible.

- Drink plenty of water. You can become dehydrated not only from sweating but also from exhaling.

- Keep moving to stay warm.

Hot weather

- Drink plenty of water to avoid dehydration.

- Walk early in the morning or late in the evening, when the temperature is at its lowest.

- Wear light, loose-fitting clothing.

- Consider going slower and for a shorter period than when the weather is cooler.

- If the humidity is more than 70 percent, watch out for heat exhaustion or heatstroke (see box). Heat and humidity interfere with the body's natural cooling process.

- If you feel any of the symptoms of heat exhaustion or heatstroke, douse yourself with water to cool down immediately. Heatstroke is potentially fatal, so act quickly.

HEAT EXHAUSTION

Stop walking immediately if you have any of these symptoms:

- Heavy sweating and cold, clammy skin
- Dizziness
- A rapid pulse
- Throbbing pressure in your head
- Chills
- Flushed appearance
- Nausea

HEATSTROKE

- Warm, dry skin with no sweating, or heavy sweating and cold, clammy skin
- Confusion and/or unconsciousness
- High fever
- A slow pulse
- Ashen or gray skin
- Low blood pressure

joan's story:
BEATING THE
BAD-WEATHER BLUES

Joan, a lifelong couch potato, was determined to change her habits. Because she worked two jobs, she didn't have much time. She did have about 45 minutes after she dropped her son off at school, however.

"I decided to walk at my son's school track each weekday morning," said Joan. "I walked every weekday for three weeks. Then on weekends my son and I rode bikes together. My clothes started to fit better, and I had more energy."

Then one Monday, it was pouring rain when she dropped her son off at school. She automatically thought, "It's raining, so I can't walk." The trouble was, it rained for four straight days. By the weekend, Joan was discouraged and upset. "I realized that I couldn't let rain be an excuse to stop walking," she said. "I bought a good raincoat that was easy to walk in and a pair of cloth sneakers that would dry quickly."

The next time it rained, Joan was ready. She now walks every day—rain or shine. If it's really cold or there is lightning, she heads to the mall and walks inside. This is one former sofa spud who won't let a little rain drown her good intentions.

Breaking the Whine Barrier

At some point in your physical-activity plan you're likely to come up with the excuses listed below for not exercising. Don't worry, that's normal whining. The important thing is that you see through these excuses to the new, active lifestyle you want. Here's what to tell yourself when these excuses arise.

I DON'T HAVE THE TIME

Hello! We're *all* busy. People make time for what really matters to them. Remember: You don't have to do your daily physical activity all at once. Three 10-minute activity sessions add up to the 30 minutes a day you need. How hard is that?

I DON'T HAVE THE ENERGY

Want energy? Then get more physical activity. It's ironic, but people who exercise regularly are rarely tired; physical activity actually *energizes* rather than depletes. Only couch potatoes are tired all the time.

I'VE NEVER LIKED TO EXERCISE

Hey, exercise is not medieval torture. It's supposed to be fun! Throw away those "no pain, no gain" images. Realize that physical activity is only movement that makes life more pleasurable: basketball, walking, gardening, tennis. It's easy to make something you enjoy a regular part of your life. Don't get in a rut: Always be willing to try something new, such as yoga, aerobic dance, hiking, bicycling, or ice skating. Think outside the box!

IT COSTS TOO MUCH

Not true. You can be physically active without buying a lot of expensive equipment. In fact, you can build activity into a normal day by simply parking farther away from work and walking part of the way, taking the stairs rather than the elevator, or walking the dog.

IT HURTS

If it hurts, slow down. You're doing too much too fast. Vary your routine enough to allow for rest between bouts of activity. When you start slowly and increase your activity bit by bit, it will feel *good*—not painful.

I'M TOO OLD

Tell that to the participants in the Senior Olympics. They're living proof that you're never too old for physical activity. Studies of seniors show that regular physical activity helps them stay independent and improves their capabilities for basic living: carrying grocery bags, doing household chores, and visiting friends.

arnold's story:
YOU'RE ONLY AS OLD AS YOU THINK

"At seventy years old, I felt older than I am now," said Arnold, a 75-year-old retired military officer. "I had quit being active and let myself not only *get* old, but *feel* old."

When Arnold couldn't keep up with his great-grandchildren anymore, he decided it was time to make a change. "I started slowly," said Arnold. "At first, I just did some stretching exercises and walked a few laps around my driveway. I also began parking farther from stores so I would have to walk more."

Soon, Arnold was walking around the block. Eventually, his wife saw how much energy he had and started joining him on his walks. "My wife and I feel great and are really enjoying our 'golden years,'" said Arnold. "I think we have become more active and energetic than our children!"

I'M NOT SEEING RESULTS QUICKLY ENOUGH

Then adjust your expectations. It takes six to eight weeks to see results, but these benefits can accumulate for a year or longer as your fitness level improves. Remember that exercise is not a quick fix, something you do for a little while and then you're finished. It's like brushing your teeth. You don't brush them once and they're fine for life. You commit to brushing as a regular routine so that your teeth will stay healthy and gleaming. Relax and have fun. The results will show up in their own time—and they'll stay with you.

I'M ON THE ROAD TOO MUCH

You can find many ways to get exercise while traveling. On car trips, for example, you can take regular walking breaks at roadside parks and scenic areas. If you're flying, arrive at the airport early and explore the concourse. On business, walk instead of taking taxis when you can. On vacation, opt for walking tours when you're sightseeing. Many hotels offer fitness centers with weight-training equipment and a jogging track. Look for the swimming, golf, tennis, and sports facilities usually found at larger hotels.

I HAVE OTHER HEALTH PROBLEMS

If so, check with your doctor. We're betting your doctor will say staying active will help your condition. Whether it's high blood pressure, high blood cholesterol, diabetes, or some other chronic condition, active people are likely to stay healthier than inactive people with these same conditions.

I DON'T WANT TO GET INJURED OR HAVE A HEART ATTACK

We don't want you to either. That's why we recommend finding an activity you like and taking it very slowly. Also, wear comfortable clothing and shoes that fit. If you increase your activity slowly and gradually, it's not likely you'll be injured. As for a heart attack while exercising, that's extremely rare. When it does happen, it usually involves a person who already has a heart condition. Physical activity actually *reduces* the risk of a heart attack.

Setting Goals— and Getting Your Just Rewards

As we said in Chapter 1, you won't get far without a long-range goal. It sets your course. It gives you something to aim for, a result you'd like to see in your life. When you have your long-range goal, you can then break it up into shorter, bite-size goals.

alma's story:
DESIGNING YOUR FUTURE

Alma is in her 40s and seriously out of shape. She's a graphics designer, working at a computer for as long as 10 to 12 hours a day. Until six months ago she would go home, cook dinner, and watch television until bedtime. For years her doctor had urged her to get more exercise, lose weight, and reduce her blood cholesterol. Then during one visit, he found that she had diabetes.

"I knew I had to do something," Alma said, "so I set several goals. First, I was going to lose twenty pounds. Second, I was going to reduce my blood cholesterol to below 200. My long-term goal was to get my diabetes under control."

These were big goals, so Alma broke them up into smaller steps. "I committed to cutting down on sugar, stop eating fried foods, and have five servings of fruits and vegetables every day," she said. "Then I started my walking plan. I promised myself that I'd take three 10-minute 'walking breaks' every day at work. I decided that on Saturdays I'd walk three miles. That takes me about 45 minutes, but I listen to audiotapes and the time flies by."

Six months later, Alma has stuck with her plan for the most part. On the rare days when she doesn't, she refuses to beat herself up. She just gets back to it as soon as possible. Her next step is to leave work early on Tuesdays to take a yoga class to improve her flexibility and help reduce stress.

Today, she's well on the way to meeting her long-range goals. She's lost 12 pounds; her blood cholesterol is 195, down from 234; and her diabetes is under control. In fact, the doctor said that her lifestyle change may be what's allowing her to control her diabetes with oral medication only—no insulin shots needed!

CREATE YOUR OWN PLAN

Take a moment now to think about your long- and short-term goals. Jot them down and review them often. They'll help you stay on track.

Besides setting long- and short-term goals, it's important to create a personal reward system. It may seem silly, but it's astoundingly motivating. Think about what rewards might motivate you. They can be luxuries of any kind: new clothes, a trip, a long bubble bath, a manicure, an hour to read or listen to music, dinner out at a new restaurant. Choose items or experiences you love but rarely treat yourself to.

Now list two or three long-term rewards and six or seven short-term—weekly—rewards.

haley's story:
REWARD YOURSELF

"I had exercised faithfully until I started to get bored," said Haley, a dress designer. "I then slowly began to let other things interfere with exercising.

"I started trying different exercises, but it didn't work," she said. "Because I already had been exercising to maintain my weight and stay in shape, I wasn't seeing a noticeable difference in my appearance anymore. That made me feel that I wasn't getting a real reward out of exercising."

She started thinking of different ways to reward herself, such as a hot bath or a new pair of shoes, but that wasn't enough. "For me, a big reward was much more important than a bunch of small ones," Haley said, "so I started saving 50 cents for every half hour of exercise. I actually took the cash and kept it in a special place separate from everything else. It was my own personal money that had to be spent on something special just for me."

Seeing the money grow every week helped Haley keep herself motivated. "I had been quitting exercising after twenty minutes because I would convince myself that it was long enough," Haley said. "With my new system, if I didn't do thirty minutes of exercise, I didn't get the reward. That was a huge motivator for me."

Now Haley's working toward buying a weekend at a spa—a perfectly wonderful way to be pampered.

Your Quick-Start-into-Action Checklist

Here's how to jump-start yourself into a lifetime of physical activity. It's the easiest 11-step program you'll ever do!

__Set long-range goals. (What do you ultimately want?)

__Set small, doable short-range goals—interim steps designed to get you to your long-range goals.

__Find a buddy. You can keep each other motivated. If you need a group, find a class or a club.

__Wear comfortable shoes and clothing.

__Find at least three activities that sound like fun. Virtually all the good movers we know chose activities they really liked—and did them on a regular basis.

__Start slowly, with just 15 minutes a day. Plan your activity into your day.

__If the activity you choose is outdoors, have a backup plan for bad weather.

__Set a definite time and place and mark your calendar. You may want to walk in your neighborhood before breakfast, take a walking break at work during your lunch hour, or go to the gym after work.

__After the second week, add five minutes to your daily activity amount (20 minutes a day).

__Every week, increase your activity by five minutes a day, until you reach 30 minutes a day. (You can stop at 30 minutes a day or continue with gradual increases.) To challenge yourself as your fitness improves, slowly increase the intensity of your activity.

__Plan ways to reward yourself for making each goal. Then be sure to follow through with your reward.

If you slip, return to your plan as soon as possible. Everyone has lapses. It's part of the process. When you slip, catch yourself quickly, admit you've slipped, then go back to your new, permanent way of life. A lapse is not failure—it's just a lapse. You fail only when you don't start over.

Remember: This is a permanent part of your life—make it fun!

PERSONAL CONTRACT

For _____ [*your name here*]

Beginning _____ [*date*], I resolve to

_____

_____ [*long-range goal*].

I know that changing my life won't happen all at once, but I'll take the following small steps to achieve my goal:

_____

_____

_____

[*short-range goals—ways you plan to modify your behavior*].

As an incentive to stick with my plan, I will reward myself with each step I take toward my goal. These rewards include:

_____

_____

_____

I realize that reaching my goal will take time and perseverance. If I wander away from this plan, I will not be defeated. I will renew my commitment.

I will also enlist my friend _____[*name*] to sign this contract with me and to offer support.

_____ [*your signature*]

_____ [*your friend's signature*]

CHAPTER 4 clearing

THE AIR

how to make a u-turn on tobacco road

"NO MATTER HOW FAR
        YOU HAVE GONE ON
    THE WRONG ROAD, TURN BACK."

—TURKISH PROVERB

IN THE LATE 1950S, THE PHILIP MORRIS TOBACCO COMPANY CREATED an icon—a smoker who epitomized the fantasy of most smokers at that time. Philip Morris called him the Marlboro Man. This rugged individualist was a cowboy, living a life of freedom under the big Montana sky. He was handsome, free, and fulfilled. And, of course, he smoked Marlboros.

This ad campaign worked to make Marlboro the largest-selling brand of cigarettes in the country. However, those who bought the fantasy and lived the Marlboro life were less successful.

At least two actors who played the Marlboro Man died of lung cancer. One of them, Wayne McLaren, began working on an antismoking campaign after he was diagnosed with cancer. He starred in a television commercial that showed him in a hospital bed just before he died. In the commercial his brother says, "Lying there with all those tubes in you, how independent can you really be?"

A popular theme of ancient Greek drama avowed that tragedy is knowledge too late. At the American Heart Association, we have to agree. It's clearly too late for some of the Marlboro Men, but it's not too late for you. The day you quit, your risk of heart disease rapidly declines. One year after quitting, the risk of heart disease and stroke for people who smoked a pack a day or less is cut in half.

Congratulations on your decision to quit smoking. We're with you all the way.

---

jason's story:
"I QUIT COLD TURKEY"

As a hard-driving stockbroker, Jason thrived on the roller-coaster ride of Wall Street trading. He had smoked three packs a day for 20 years. One Monday morning, he learned that his twin brother, also a heavy smoker, had had a heart attack. The brother barely survived, needing a triple-bypass operation.

"That got my attention," Jason remembered. "I had heard all the warnings about smoking. I'm not an idiot. I just didn't think it would happen to me. I went to see my brother in the hospital. It was like looking at myself in that hospital bed. When I got back to New York, I called a stop-smoking program and enrolled. I was nervous but determined. I quit cold turkey. It was hard, especially at work, where every cell cries out for a cigarette. But I was highly motivated. There comes a day when you know it's cigarettes or you. I chose me. That was more than 25 years ago."

Why **Smoking** Is Playing with Fire

When urged to quit smoking, people often say, "Well, I don't have too many other vices." With a vice like this, you don't need *any* others. Smoking alone will do you in. Smoking is the greatest cause of preventable death in our society. It directly accounts for more than 400,000 deaths a year in the United States.

A smoker's risk of heart attack is more than twice that of a nonsmoker. If a smoker does have a heart attack, he or she is more likely to die—and to die suddenly (within an hour). Because smoking can lead to high blood pressure, a smoker has three times a nonsmoker's risk of stroke.

---

jonathan's story:
SMOKING IS NOT REALLY COOL

"My whole life was planned around smoking," said Jonathan, a saxophone player in a nightclub. "Just to go to our neighbor's barbecue was a major production. I had to have plenty of cigarettes, a lighter, and matches in case the lighter didn't work. And extra cigarettes—just in case. It was an obsession."

Jonathan started smoking when he joined

the army. It was easy to pick up the habit because free cigarettes were handed out to soldiers. "Everyone smoked, so I started," said Jonathan. "It didn't take long to get hooked. The ads say smoking is glamorous and sexy, and if you don't like it, you can always quit. That's a laugh."

When Jonathan began to hear about the health risks of smoking, he decided to quit. But quitting wasn't as easy as the ads suggested. Finally, he got a nudge in the right direction—but it was almost too late.

His wife was driving him to the club late one afternoon when Jonathan started feeling weak and dizzy. His wife pulled over to the side of the street, came around, and opened his door.

"My right arm went limp, and my cigarette fell on the ground," he said. "That was the last cigarette I ever smoked." Although Jonathan's right arm was paralyzed, he recovered from his stroke. He had a special sax made and has taught himself to play it with one hand. He has also dedicated himself to educating people about cigarette smoking and strokes. He always urges people to quit smoking before they have no choice.

Of course, lung cancer is another major possibility for smokers. In fact, smoking causes 87 percent of all lung cancer. Lung cancer kills more women than breast cancer. Since 1950, lung cancer deaths among women in the United States have increased 500 percent. In addition to lung cancer, smoking also contributes to cancer of the mouth, throat, esophagus, gastrointestinal tract, urinary tract, cervix, and stomach.

Smokers are also prone to develop other fatal lung diseases, such as emphysema, a chronic degenerative disease that makes breathing increasingly difficult. With emphysema, the walls between the lungs' tiny air sacs break down. The tissue loses its elasticity, so the lungs can't expand and contract normally. Each breath becomes harder, and the person becomes progressively weaker due to lack of oxygen. Eventually, even minor physical activity is impossible. At the end, even a tank of oxygen is no help. The lungs are just like sacks—unable to move air or oxygen.

If you're a woman who smokes, you can expect even more problems. For example, if you smoke and use oral contraceptives, you have a higher risk of developing blood clots and having a heart attack. Your risk of stroke also dramatically increases.

Smoking during pregnancy can result in a baby with low birth weight, plus an increased risk of spontaneous abortion, premature birth, or even the baby's death. Exposure to smoke can retard growth of the fetus, adversely affecting the child's long-term growth and intellectual development.

Later in a woman's life, smoking can cause premature menopause. Smoking can lower estrogen levels, increasing the risk of osteoporosis.

What Happens When You Put Out the Flames

The minute you quit smoking, your chances of getting smoking-related diseases begins to decline.

Within 48 hours

Pulse rate drops
Temperature of hands and feet increases
Carbon monoxide level in blood drops to normal
Oxygen level in blood increases to normal
Chance of having a heart attack decreases
Nerve endings start regrowing
Ability to smell and taste is enhanced

Within a few months

Circulation improves
Walking becomes easier
Lung function improves

Within one year

Coughing, sinus congestion, and fatigue decrease
Shortness of breath goes away
Risk of coronary heart disease is cut in half

Within three years

For people who smoked a pack a day or less, risk of death from heart disease or stroke is almost the same as for people who never smoked

At ten years

Risk of lung cancer drops by 50 percent

At fifteen years

Risk of all smoking-related deaths decreases to that of people who have never smoked

elisa's story:
HOOKED

As a salesperson, Elisa worked night and day. She traveled a lot, exhibited at trade shows, and had many meetings over dinner and drinks. Since all her peers smoked, Elisa took up the habit.

"I was always tense when I was preparing a presentation. I smoked to relax. I smoked to lose weight. I smoked to look hip," she remembered. "I always thought I could quit anytime, but it wasn't long before I began chain smoking when I was alone—not just while working or out at night. I couldn't go anywhere or do anything without a cigarette. If I found myself without one, I'd get panicky. I'd bum cigarettes, smoke butts, walk blocks out of my way just to get a smoke. I was totally hooked."

She planned to quit smoking when she reached age 30, but then she was unable to quit. "I got some therapy and learned I had been using cigarettes to blot out all my insecurities and fears. I smoked so I wouldn't feel so scared and out of it. It took about a year, but I finally quit for good. And I now know that I can do a great job without cigarettes."

Calling It Quits

In some ways, quitting smoking may be the hardest thing you ever do. Almost 80 percent of all smokers who try to stop smoking fail on their first attempt. In fact, most smokers quit several times before they finally succeed.

It's important to remember that quitting smoking is a *process,* and relapses are natural. Most people who've quit say that the process is somewhat like breaking down a door: You may not be able to get through on the first try, but the door will be a little weaker. Hitting the door again makes it even weaker. If you keep hitting it, eventually it will cave in—and you'll be on the other side.

REASONS FOR PACKING IT IN

Here are some of the most common reasons for stopping the smoking habit:

"To avoid having a heart attack or a stroke."

"To stop coughing and prevent lung diseases."

"To help my baby be healthy."

"To set a good example for my kids."

"To have more energy."

"To be able to walk or run farther."

"To taste my food again."

"To save money."

You may have other reasons as well. Write your reasons on an index card and post it on the bathroom mirror, the refrigerator, the sun visor in your car, or wherever you will see it, to remind yourself why you're quitting.

YOU HAVE NOTHING TO FEAR BUT FEAR ITSELF

When you come right down to it, the fear of quitting includes the fear of withdrawal symptoms, gaining weight, nicotine cravings, loss of friendships and support from your smoking friends, general anxiety, restlessness, and irritability.

Fortunately, you can greatly reduce the severity of withdrawal symptoms, minimize your weight gain, and effectively cope with the psychological difficulties of quitting. We will show you how.

CONSTANT CRAVINGS

When you start the process of quitting, you'll feel three main urges to smoke.

Physical urge

The urge to smoke is real because of your body's hunger for nicotine. You'll experience real physical withdrawal symptoms, including light-headedness, sleepiness, or headaches. Fortunately, symptoms will go away within a week or two. Unfortunately, the physical urge to smoke will continue for a long time, gradually weakening until it's undetectable.

Whenever you get the urge to smoke, stop what you're doing and *time the urge*. You'll find that it lasts just a minute or two. Try to hold out until the urge passes. In time, these urges will get shorter and weaker, until one day they are no more than a fleeting thought.

Feeling of being deprived

This is difficult to shake. That's because you've used cigarettes for all sorts of reasons: to deaden hunger pangs, to cope with awkward social situations, to reward yourself for a job well done, to ease the pain of loneliness or insecurity, or to comfort yourself and feel good. Without these aids, you'll feel deprived, even miserable. The key here is to *substitute other behaviors* in these situations.

For example, perhaps you normally light up a cigarette when you feel frustrated, worried, or anxious. Now, instead of allowing smoking to deflect these emotions, you'll want to learn to accept them, feel them, and express them. You may be more irritable for a few weeks. You can help counteract this problem with breathing exercises, meditation, or walking or other physical activities, and by building lots of fun into your life. These activities will help you deal with the frustrations and anxieties of life— without smoking.

Smoking out of habit

This happens because your mind and body are programmed to want cigarettes at certain times. For example, you may crave a cigarette in the morning, after meals, with coffee or alcohol, or when you watch television. This programmed response becomes automatic.

Remind yourself that *you're not a slave*. You can change any habit, including this one. You trained yourself to need cigarettes at certain times to make yourself feel normal. You can now retrain yourself to feel normal without them. You're the same person you were before you started smoking.

---

leroy's story:
"I CRAVED CIGARETTES"

Leroy teaches fifth grade. His warmth, energy, and offbeat sense of humor have made him popular with students. In fact, he's been voted best homeroom teacher in his school three years in a row.

"When I think about it, it's amazing that I was able to teach as well as I did, get this kind of response and support, and still hide a two-pack-a-day smoking habit," said Leroy. "I knew I had to quit, but my body craved cigarettes. I'd stop class on some pretense, tell them to work a problem or write something, then race down to the teachers' lounge and smoke half a cigarette, just to stay sane. When I had to, I went into the janitor's closet. It was crazy."

Leroy tried to quit many times, but he always started again. Ultimately, his addiction got so far out of control that he simply couldn't hide it. His unscheduled smoking breaks began to draw attention. Finally, the principal spoke with him.

"That was humiliating," said Leroy. "I'm a capable person. I worked my way through school, I'm an award-winning teacher, but I just couldn't discipline myself to quit smoking. Lucky for me, the school system has a program for addictions. I got some help. I also used nicotine gum to help me quit. I haven't smoked for six years now. I count it as a miracle that probably saved my life."

How to Beat the Tar Out of Smoking Urges

When you have a sudden, strong urge to smoke, it can often take you by surprise. To give yourself a fighting chance, it's smart to plan your response. The following tried-and-true urge-control measures can help you stay in the winner's circle:

Stop what you're doing when the urge starts.

Move to a different room.

Walk around for one to two minutes.

Breathe deeply. Breathe in slowly while you count to five, then breathe out slowly while you count to five.

Squirt your throat with a breath freshener. It will help replace that scratchy feeling you miss.

Brush your teeth.

Use mouthwash.

Call a friend or friends for support. Write their numbers here:

Friend #1: _____

Friend #2: _____

Friend #3: _____

Chew something to keep your mouth busy: carrot sticks, radishes, celery, sugarless gum or breath mints, jelly beans, or low-fat popcorn.

Drink something cold.

List all the drawbacks of smoking and all the benefits of quitting. Imagine how great you'll feel as a nonsmoker.

Practice relaxation.

Time the urge to smoke. At first it lasts a minute or two. As the weeks go by, these urges will weaken until you hardly notice them.

AN OUNCE OF PREVENTION

Luckily, you can actually reduce the number and strength of the urges you get. Here's how.

DON'T LET YOURSELF GET TOO TIRED OR HUNGRY

Eat three to six nutritious meals a day, and have non-fat or low-fat snacks on hand if you need them. Here are some ideas:

Small sandwiches
Cut-up vegetables
Bread or bagels
Breadsticks
Nonfat or low-fat muffins
Popcorn
Fruit or fruit juice
Nonfat or low-fat yogurt
Pretzels
Angel food cake
Marshmallows
Fig bars
Cereal
Soda crackers
Nonfat or low-fat frozen yogurt
Diet soft drinks

CUT DOWN ON COFFEE AND TEA

Try this for a few weeks if these drinks trigger your need to smoke. If coffee and tea don't make you want to smoke, continue to drink them. If you give up coffee or other forms of caffeine at the same time you quit smoking, you may have two strong addictions to fight at the same time.

RELAX

It's vital to quitting. Use biofeedback, meditation, warm baths, music, needlework, stress-reducing activities, exercise—whatever it takes to get and stay relaxed.

COUNT CASH

How much do you spend every day on cigarettes?

Write it here: _____

Now, multiply by 100 and write it here: _____

This is what you'll save in just over three months when you're not smoking. Think of something fun you could do with this money.

GET SOME TYPE OF EXERCISE EVERY DAY

Whether it's walking, swimming, or a pickup game of basketball, one of the best things you can do to kick the smoking habit is to exercise daily. Why? Because physical activity reduces stress, calms you, cuts depression, helps you pass the time, helps control your appetite, burns calories, and puts more fun in your life. Fun is the operative term. Find at least one type of physical activity you really like and "just do it"—every day. For a list of fun activities, check out page 121 in the section on physical activity.

SPOIL YOURSELF

That's right, you heard us. See a new movie, visit old friends, have a picnic in the park, attend a sporting event, buy some beautiful music, get a massage, start a creative project, eat out at a good restaurant, take naps, go on a fishing trip, or throw a party. Whatever it takes to add fun to your life, *do it*. When the going gets tough, you may feel your life is empty without cigarettes. These fun activities and pleasures will show you that life can actually be full and fun—without cigarettes.

---

sheldon's story:
GUILT IS NOT ENOUGH

Every time Sheldon lit up a cigarette, he felt guilty. As sales manager of a company that made exercise equipment, he felt like a total hypocrite. More than anybody, he knew the health risks of smoking as well as the benefits of exercise. And although he did exercise, he simply could not quit smoking.

"I started smoking in Vietnam. As a soldier, you had hours of total boredom punctuated by moments of sheer terror," said Sheldon. "Everyone smoked just to get through it. When I got back to the States, I tried halfheartedly to quit, but couldn't."

Sheldon had been a jock in high school, and working out was second nature to him. He and a buddy teamed up to create one of the biggest names in exercise equipment. As the company grew, so did Sheldon's guilt. But he refused to get help. "I was stubborn. Wouldn't take help from anybody. Wanted to do everything myself," said Sheldon. "Quitting a seventeen-year smoking habit was no exception. So I signed up for a month-long survival course taught in the desert wilderness area of Big Bend National Park. And I didn't take any cigarettes."

The first week was hellish. Sheldon was desperate for a cigarette. The urge never left him. He was so irritable that the instructor wanted to kill him, and so did the other students. In fact, Sheldon said he would have paid them to do it. It was that bad.

"After about ten days, it began to ease up," said Sheldon. "I hardly felt any urge to smoke after the second week. After the third week, I was home free. At the end of the course, the instructor gave us each a T-shirt that read I Survived the Big Bend Desert Survival Training Course. It had a picture of a vulture on the front. We all laughed. Desert survival is no picnic. But my real survival feat that month was quitting smoking. By comparison, dragging yourself across the desert with no water is a piece of cake."

Smoke and Mirrors: What **Really** Makes You Want to Light Up?

To quit smoking for good, you'll need to track down exactly what situations create the craving to smoke. You can locate these trigger situations by taking the test below. It will help you determine how confident you feel about resisting the urge to smoke in typical situations.

QUIT-SMOKING CONFIDENCE QUESTIONNAIRE

Read through the situations below. If you're absolutely certain you won't smoke in that situation, write "10" in the space to the right. If you have no confidence at all, write "0." On a scale of 1 to 10, rate your *ability to resist* smoking in each situation.

1. When you feel bored or depressed _____

2. When you see others smoking _____

3. When you want to relax or rest _____

4. When you just want to sit back and enjoy a cigarette _____

5. When you are watching television _____

6. When you are driving or riding in a car _____

7. When you have finished a meal or snack _____

8. When you feel frustrated, worried, upset, tense, nervous, angry, anxious, or annoyed _____

9. When you want to snack but don't want to gain weight _____

10. When you need more energy or can't concentrate _____

11. When someone offers you a cigarette _____

12. When you are drinking coffee or tea _____

13. When you are in a situation in which alcohol is involved _____

14. When you feel smoking is part of your self-image _____

If you gave yourself 3 or less on any of these situations, they're especially risky. You'll want to focus on them first.

Below, you'll find Action Plans to help you in each situation. Copy your confidence scores onto these Action Plans and use these strategies in high-risk situations. In fact, no matter how high your confidence score, it's a good idea to review each situation and its strategy. You never know when temptation will strike.

SMOKING SITUATION ACTION PLANS

When certain situations arise, the urge to smoke seems almost overwhelming. But a plan of action can help you avoid temptation. Here are action plans for the 14 most common smoking situations.

1. When you feel bored or depressed

Confidence Rating _____

- *Keep moving.* Take a quick walk around the block or even to another room. Amazingly, it will help change your mood.

- *Can we talk?* Even if you don't feel like it, call a friend or find someone at work or home to talk to. It will help ease the boredom.

- *I'm outta here.* Make vacation plans or plan a fun project or activity.

- *The great escapes.* Find something interesting to read or treat yourself to a video. It will take your mind off your depression.

- *Get in the game.* Don't let yourself get bored. Take on a project you've been putting off, or fill your time with fun activities such as going to the movies, bike rides, sports events, eating out, gardening, fishing, or visiting friends.

- *This too will pass.* Instead of focusing on your depression, say, "What I'm feeling is normal, and it will pass."

- *Yuck.* Ask yourself if it would really cheer you up to stick poison in your mouth and set fire to it.

- List your own ideas: _____
_____
_____

2. When you see others smoking

Confidence Rating _____

- *Avoidance therapy.* For the first few weeks, do your best to keep away from all smokers. Even if they don't offer you cigarettes, they'll remind you of your old smoking life.

- *It pays to advertise.* If you can't avoid a smoker, be sure to mention you've quit.

- *No guts, no glory.* Allow yourself to feel a little smug. After all, *you've* managed to stop.

- *Just say no.* If you know you'll be seeing friends who still smoke, practice ahead of time saying, "No, thanks. I've quit!"

- *Clear the air.* Always choose the nonsmoking sections in restaurants.

- List your own ideas: _____
_____
_____

3. When you want to relax or rest

Confidence Rating   ____

- *Chill out.* Lie back in a comfortable chair and relax for 10 to 15 minutes. Use a tape or restful music if you like.

- *Quick fix.* If you don't have time to fully relax, do a mini version: breathe in deeply and slowly, while you silently count to five. Then breathe out slowly, counting to five again.

- *Walking papers.* Take a short walk just to relax.

- *Take your time.* Set aside at least 30 minutes each day just for you, and use it to relax.

- *Child's play.* Take up some soothing hobbies, such as needlework, jigsaw puzzles, or model making.

- *Rest assured.* Find activities that relax you—meditation, concerts, gardening—then do them regularly.

- List your own ideas: _____

  _____

  _____

4. When you just want to sit back and enjoy a cigarette

Confidence Rating _____

- *Find alternatives.* Okay. So cigarettes were your reward. Find something else. Try five or ten minutes of complete relaxation.

- *Spoil yourself instead.* For a few weeks, arrange to watch your favorite television shows, listen to your favorite music, and do the things that make you feel happy.

- *Yum.* Treat yourself to your favorite food. Eat it slowly and savor it!

- *Anticipation.* Plan ahead to handle those times when your body automatically wants a cigarette. For example, if you used to smoke after a meal, plan to get up from the table as soon as you've finished eating—and do something else!

- *Break a habit*. If you normally smoked in a certain place, such as your favorite easy chair, sit somewhere else for a while. It will help you disassociate smoking and location.

- List your own ideas: _____
_____
_____

---

carol's story:
SURPRISE ENDING

After 20 years as a pack-a-day smoker, Carol made the decision to quit. But her reason for doing so was unusual: She and her husband, Ron, wanted to run the New York City Marathon together—just to say they could do it. Although Carol was athletic, she had never run a marathon. She realized during the training that she'd have to quit smoking in order to have the endurance it would take to stay with him for the 26-mile ordeal.

"I wasn't quitting cigarettes for good, mind you. Just until I finished the marathon. Then I planned to smoke again," said Carol. "I didn't worry about the health risks or any of that stuff. I just wanted to be able to compete. I wanted to cross the finish line at the New York City Marathon with my husband."

Carol did all the smart things. She stayed away from friends who smoked, avoided parties, and kept raw carrots in her desk at work to munch on when the craving got serious. Ron admitted he was astounded. He honestly thought she wouldn't be able to do it. "I *know* Carol," Ron said. "Smoking and all the paraphernalia that goes with it are a huge part of her life. The problem of what to do with her hands alone, I figured, would be insurmountable!"

But Carol did quit smoking. Then she and Ron trained for seven months. Finally, the day of the New York City Marathon arrived. Their son and daughter were standing by with Carol's parents as Carol and Ron received their numbers and lined up among the thousands of participants. A little more than four hours after the starting gun, an exhausted but elated Carol finally made it across the finish line just behind her husband. When she arrived, she had a real surprise: She had no desire to resume smoking.

"After all that training and running, I had completely lost my interest in cigarettes," said Carol. "That was seven years ago. I never think about it."

5. When you're watching television

Confidence Rating ___

- *Glad hands.* Find something to do with your hands when you're watching television, such as sewing, knitting, putting photos in albums, or building a model airplane.

- *Television trivia.* Get up and stretch during commercials or walk around the house.

- *Lip service.* Give your mouth something to do other than smoke. Sip water with lemon juice or eat plain popcorn (made without oil).

- *Lose your television.* If television gives you serious urges, watch less of it for a while. Instead, listen to music, play board games, read books, or get out of the house.

- *Video R and R.* Practice relaxing while you watch television.

- List your own ideas: _____
_____
_____

6. When you're driving or riding in a car

Confidence Rating ___

- *Toss the ashtray.* You heard us: Remove your car's ashtray. Leave it out of your car, or wash it and put it back with a photo of someone you love in it.

- *A breath of fresh air.* Roll down the window and breathe deeply.

- *Music major.* Change the radio station or put in a new tape. Turn up the volume and sing along.

- *Crunchy munchies.* Keep gum or low-calorie snacks in the car.

- *Smoke-free zone.* If you're riding with others, ask them not to smoke.

- *Smell-o-vision.* Look at smokers in other cars. Imagine what their cars will smell like for the rest of the day.

- List your own ideas: _____

  _____

  _____

7. When you have finished a meal or snack

Confidence Rating _____

- *Outta sight.* Don't linger at the table. Get up and do something else.

- *Busy mouth.* Nibble on a low-calorie food (carrots, breadsticks, fruit) so you can keep on eating after you've finished the main meal.

- *Change of taste.* Chew gum or a strong mint right after eating.

- *Fresh is best.* Brush your teeth. Then use a mouthwash or spray the back of your mouth with a breath freshener.

- *Avoid temptation.* In restaurants, always sit in the nonsmoking section.

- *Ethnic excitement.* Try new restaurants, especially those with spicy foods—the cuisines of India, Mexico, Thailand, or parts of China are great choices. These foods can give you new taste sensations that may help you forget the desire for a cigarette.

- *A walk on the outside.* If you're in a restaurant, get up and take a two-minute stroll outside after you've eaten.

- *Talk therapy.* If you're alone, telephone a friend as soon as you finish eating.

- List your own ideas: _____

  _____

  _____

8. When you feel frustrated, worried, upset, tense, nervous, angry, anxious, or annoyed

Confidence Rating   ____

- *Hold on*. You may have used cigarettes to deflect many of your emotions. Now that you don't have that shield, they're hitting you with full force. Be patient. It may be rough for a few weeks, but you will adjust.

- *Don't fight the feeling*. Let your feelings wash over you. Don't fight them; rather, take the time and effort to communicate them genuinely, but with kindness.

- *Storm warning*. Alert your family and friends that you may be more irritable for a few weeks. Ask them not to take it personally.

- *Cool down*. If you feel very irritable, count to ten to calm yourself down.

- *Let go*. Take time to relax deeply every day. When you feel tense or anxious, try the instant relaxation exercise described in situation number three.

- *Move around*. Walk down the hall, around the yard, or around the block.

- *Playtime*. Try to keep your life stocked with good times. Make specific plans to entertain yourself.

- List your own ideas: _____

  _____

  _____

9. When you want to snack but don't want to gain weight

Confidence Rating ____

- *Snack attack.* Plan ahead for foods that you can eat without guilt, such as vegetables, fruits, popcorn, breads, and sugar-free candies.

- *Calorie counter.* Carry some low calorie food with you at all times. Stash some in places where you spend a lot of time, such as your car or workplace.

- *More than you can chew.* Carry sugarless gum with you. Keep a selection of different flavors handy.

- *Fake it till you make it.* If your lips miss the feel of a cigarette, experiment with objects such as drinking straws cut into cigarette-size lengths.

- *Good eats.* Choose low-fat foods and read the labels on prepared foods to make sure you're getting good nutrition without a lot of calories.

- List your own ideas: _____
_____
_____

conrad's story:
ATTITUDE ADJUSTMENT

"I lived on caffeine and nicotine. There's big money in my business, but you have to be first with the best," said Conrad, a software developer for an internationally known video-game manufacturer. "My cup of coffee and pack of cigarettes were always right next to my computer."

About every two years, Conrad would get worried about lung cancer and try to quit smoking. When he did, he was a nightmare to be around: anxious, irritable, hyperactive, jittery, unable to sleep, and unable to concentrate on anything. He convinced himself that he couldn't create award-winning video games without cigarettes.

"I was in my forties. Still figured I was bullet-proof. Nothing fazed me until my boss, Jim, had a heart attack at work," said Conrad. "People were running and screaming. Jim looked gray. I thought he was dead. He did make it, but that scene changed my attitude overnight. Jim smoked too, and I can't count the times he and I were at my computer trying to work out a problem, smoking away like two faulty stoves. Before Jim's heart attack, I was a real martyr when I tried to quit smoking. If I went three days without a cigarette, I thought I deserved the Nobel Prize. But no more. I got serious, got help, and quit. I did it because I *wanted* to. In fact, there's no other reason to do it, because nothing else works."

---

10. When you need more energy or can't concentrate

Confidence Rating   ____

- *Out to lunch.* Tell yourself that just because you feel slow doesn't mean you *are* slow. You're missing the artificial stimulation of cigarettes. For a few months your brain may feel like it's in low gear. You may even suspect that you've lost some brain cells. You haven't. When you need them, they'll snap to attention.

- *Stay focused.* If you have an important job to do, leave plenty of time for it. To maintain your concentration, you may need to work in short bursts.

- *Go with the flow.* Appreciate your new, temporary dopiness. Sit back with some really dumb movies or sitcoms. Take naps. Hibernate.

- *Can-do attitude.* Remind yourself that *you can do it!* If you really need energy, you'll get it.

- *Wake up.* Stay alert with a brief walk.

- List your own ideas: _____
  _____
  _____

11. When someone offers you a cigarette

Confidence Rating _____

- *Quiet on the set.* Hey, this is your big moment! Some ex-smokers pray for someone to offer them a cigarette, especially if there's a big audience. Prepare your speech about having quit so that you can relish your moment of stardom.

- *Steer clear.* On the other hand, you may prefer to avoid this situation. Even if you think your willpower is strong, it's best not to test it for the first few months. That's why you should mention that you've quit as soon as you see that pack come out.

- *Lose the losers.* If certain people persist in offering you cigarettes, you'll know who your secret enemies are. Time to make *real* friends.

- *Birds of a feather.* You know where the smokers are likely to gather at work and at play. Avoid those places for a while.

- List your own ideas: _____

_____

_____

12. When you're drinking coffee or tea

Confidence Rating _____

- *Taste test.* Use the taste of the coffee or tea to make your mouth happy. Roll it around and enjoy it.

- *Make a new plan, Stan.* Change your coffee or tea routine. For example, sit in a different chair, drink from a different cup, or drink standing up.

- *Coffee break.* Try new flavors of coffee or tea, and imagine trying to describe the taste. Hold each sip in your mouth while silently counting to three.

- *Move your mouth.* Nibble on toast, crackers, or other low-calorie food.

- *Hit and run.* Drink your coffee faster than usual, then get up and do something else.

- List your own ideas: _____

_____

_____

13. When you're in a situation where alcohol is involved

Confidence Rating _____

- *You booze, you lose.* Alcohol can wreck your willpower, so be on your guard whenever it's around. Try not to drink in situations where cigarettes are easy to get.

- *Glass ceiling.* Ideally, don't drink alcohol. Drink fruit juice or carbonated water instead. If you do drink, limit yourself to one drink a day.

- *Take steps to get help.* If you feel you have a drinking problem and find it's really hard to cut down to one drink a day, get help. Call your local chapter of Alcoholics Anonymous and ask if they have nonsmoking meetings in your area.

- *Think before you drink.* If you must be in situations where alcohol and cigarettes are present, plan ahead. Stay close to nonsmokers, ask for a nonalcoholic drink, find low-fat snacks to chew, and keep your hands and mouth busy.

- List your own ideas: _____
  _____
  _____

14. When you feel smoking is part of your self-image

- *New rules.* Maybe it was bad luck that you grew up at a time when smoking supposedly made you look sophisticated. But wake up and smell the fresh air: Smoking is out.

- *Too cool.* Remember Yul Brynner and John Wayne, two of the famous stars who popularized smoking in the movies? Today they're dead from lung cancer—too high a price to pay to look cool.

- *Mas macho?* Perhaps you feel it's macho to smoke. Trust us, it's much more macho to quit.

- *The new you.* Want a cool self-image? Lose the cigarettes. Then shop carefully for some new clothes that make a statement about your new self.

- List your own ideas: _____
_____
_____

shirley's story:
"I WAS TOTALLY ALONE"

The week before their 28th wedding anniversary, Shirley's husband left her for a younger woman. Shirley was so shocked that she just sat for days. She didn't work for a week. Then one day Shirley, who had smoked for 33 years, saw an ad on television for smoking-cessation classes. She needed to get her mind off her husband, so she decided to take on a new project—quitting smoking.

This was a tall order. Shirley could barely move without a cigarette. She smoked while she was talking on the phone, working at the computer, having a discussion, enjoying a party, driving to the mall. If she could have smoked in the shower, she would have.

"I was totally alone for the first time in my life," said Shirley. "The quitting process was hard, but I had a lot of time to think. I thought of lots of good things I could do for myself, changes I could make to get on my feet again."

Shirley joined the smoking-cessation class and attended weekly. She got a makeover. She joined a health club, went on a diet, and lost 18 pounds.

"My friends were astonished," she said. "I changed in a big way. I took myself seriously for the first time ever. I started feeling good and looking good. Today, I'm a new person. And I'm a nonsmoker."

Getting **Help** from Nicotine Gum, Patches, Inhalers, and Drugs

If you smoked a pack a day for 20 years, taking 10 puffs on each cigarette, that amounts to nearly 1.5 million puffs. If you associate these hits of nicotine with pleasant events and the relief of tension, you'll have a powerful psychological dependency on this drug.

At the same time, nicotine is highly addictive. Some studies show that it's as hard to break yourself from nicotine addiction as from heroin. For these reasons, you may need to wean yourself off nicotine using nicotine gum, patches, inhalers, or drugs. Which one of these therapies is best? It depends on your temperament and the level of your addiction. Here's the story on nicotine therapies:

- *Nicotine gum.* Usually prescribed in 2- and 4-milligram doses, nicotine gum is available over the counter. About 23 percent of users

are able to quit within six months; 16 to
18 percent, within one year. If combined with
other behavioral strategies such as counseling,
family support, stress reduction, exercise, and
relapse prevention, 29 percent of users quit
within one year.

- *Nicotine patch.* Available since 1991, the patch
  is similar in effect to nicotine gum. Prescribed
  in varying doses, usually 5 to 21 milligrams,
  the patch is used over a period of about eight
  weeks. The quit rates are similar to those with
  nicotine gum, with a 26 percent success rate at
  six months.

- *Nicotine inhalers and sprays.* Nicotine inhalers
  provide a vapor that delivers about the same
  amount of nicotine as the gum. Quit rates
  at the end of six months are between 17 and
  21 percent. Nicotine nasal spray releases
  1 milligram of nicotine through the nasal
  membranes and takes effect quickly—within
  10 minutes of use. At first, you use it one or
  two times an hour, up to a maximum of
  40 milligrams a day. From 23 to 27 percent of
  users quit after one year.

- *Bupropion hydrochloride.* Originally developed as
  an antidepressant, this drug was found to help
  smokers quit. Studies show that given in doses
  of 150 or 300 milligrams a day, bupropion
  hydrochloride helps smokers quit better than a

placebo. In fact, bupropion hydrochloride at 330 milligrams a day was found to help maintain abstinence through 26 weeks. At the end of six months, 27 percent of users had successfully quit. The combination of bupropion hydrochloride and the nicotine patch is also effective.

Combining the various nicotine therapies cited above has resulted in six-month quit rates as high as 40 percent. Are you a good candidate for these therapies? Take the nicotine addiction test below to find out.

NICOTINE ADDICTION TEST

Here's one way to determine whether you'd bene-fit from nicotine gum, patches, or other therapies. Check the statements that are true for you.

__When I can't smoke, I crave a cigarette.

__I smoke my first cigarette within 30 minutes of waking up in the morning.

__I smoke at least one pack a day.

__I find it hard to keep from smoking for more than a few hours.

__When I'm sick enough to stay in bed, I still smoke.

If you checked two or more, it's likely that nico-tine therapies can help you. Of course, you'll want to discuss it with your doctor to make sure.

phil's story:
"THE DOCTOR TOLD ME TO QUIT"

Phil owned a popular deli in Chicago. His customers came in to experience Phil's quick wit as much as the corned beef on rye. He and his wife each smoked two and a half packs a day. One day he noticed a cough that wouldn't go away. His wife urged a trip to the doctor, but Phil put it off. Finally his wife won the battle, and Phil went for a checkup. Phil had a bronchitis-like condition that was irritating his lungs and threatening to get worse. The doctor advised Phil to quit smoking.

"That was the same as a death sentence to me," said Phil. "Smoking was a huge part of my life. I didn't know how to function without it. I had this craving, this desperate need to get a specific kind of feeling in my chest—and only smoking delivers it. I *had* to smoke. Yet with this lung condition, I *had* to quit."

Phil was on the ropes. He looked into stop-smoking classes but didn't like the regimented approach. He asked a dozen others how they quit, and he got a dozen different stories. "There's a stop-smoking story for every ex-smoker out there," said Phil. "I didn't know what to do. Then I heard about nicotine gum. At the time, it was relatively new, and I was skeptical. It seemed too easy. Still, I decided to give it a try. The amazing thing is, the gum satisfied that craving in my chest. I realized then that it was the nicotine addiction that caused that feeling. It took me a few tries, but I finally quit. I'll tell you, it would have been impossible without the nicotine gum. I couldn't have stopped without it. No way."

More good news: Phil's wife eventually quit too—using nicotine gum.

NICOTINE GUM: DON'T BITE OFF MORE THAN YOU CAN CHEW

By far the most popular nicotine therapy is the chewing gum. It's easy and convenient, and it works. On the other hand, nicotine gum is not for everyone. It shouldn't be used by:

- Nonsmokers

- Pregnant or nursing mothers

- People with active temporomandibular joint syndrome (TMJ) or any condition aggravated by constant chewing

- People with angina

- Anyone who has recently had a heart attack

- Anyone with a cardiac arrhythmia (irregular heartbeat)

- Anyone with a history of coronary heart disease, periodontal disease, hyperthyroidism, Raynaud's disease, insulin-dependent diabetes, high blood pressure, peptic ulcers, or inflammation of the esophagus

CHEW ON THIS

If you think nicotine gum will work for you, buy it well before your quit date. Because it's sensitive to light and heat, store it in the refrigerator (but not the freezer) until you're ready to use it. When you quit, go cold turkey. This may seem harsh, but studies show that quitting all at once is more successful than gradually cutting down.

Don't actually use the gum until you've quit smoking. Remember that nicotine hits the brain more quickly when you smoke it than when you chew the gum. If you smoke again after starting the gum, you'll likely trigger stronger urges and cravings for the quick hits you get from smoking. *Warning: Don't smoke once you've started using the gum. It can be dangerous because you're getting a double dose of nicotine.*

HOW TO USE NICOTINE GUM

The night before your quit day, throw out all your cigarettes. Get them out of your house, car, coat pocket, and purse. As soon as you get out of bed the morning of your quit day, start using the nicotine gum. Most people make the mistake of using too few pieces of gum at first. Start out by chewing one piece of gum per hour for 12 hours each day. If the cravings are still too great, increase the amount to two pieces per hour.

Avoid the temptation of thinking that you'll chew a piece of gum only when you get a craving. That's too little, too late. The nicotine in the gum may take 30 minutes to build up to high enough levels in your blood to quell the cravings. A cigarette will give you that level in seven seconds. Don't risk it. Keep your nicotine level high enough to fight off these cravings, especially in the beginning.

Be sure to chew slowly. If you chew quickly, you may experience side effects, including light-headedness, nausea, vomiting, jaw muscle ache, hiccups, or throat and mouth irritation. Here's how to do it:

- Chew the nicotine gum very slowly until you sense a peppery taste or feel a slight tingling sensation in your mouth. When you do feel this, place the gum between your cheek and gum and let it sit for a minute. The tingling sensation should subside.

- Continue chewing slowly until these sensations return. Then stop chewing again and place the gum in a different part of your mouth.

- Repeat this chewing and holding technique for 30 minutes. That's how long it takes to release most of the nicotine in the gum.

- Chew one piece of gum per hour for 12 hours each day for the first month after you quit smoking. Do it even when you think you don't need it. That's because cravings and withdrawal symptoms can reappear with surprising intensity, especially during stressful times. When that happens, you must be ready.

- It's possible to overdose on nicotine gum if you chew several pieces at the same time or in rapid succession, so remember to chew *slowly* and *deliberately*.

- *Important:* Never chew more than 30 pieces of 2-milligram gum in any one day.

- When you've quit smoking, don't stop using nicotine gum abruptly. Instead, reduce it gradually to avoid experiencing withdrawal symptoms from the gum itself. The following schedule will let you down easy.

GETTING OFF NICOTINE GUM

	NUMBER OF SMOKE-FREE WEEKS						
	3	4	5	6	7	8	9
PIECES PER DAY	26-30	21-25	16-20	11-15	6-10	1-5	0
	21-25	17-21	13-17	9-13	5-9	1-5	0
	16-20	13-17	10-14	7-11	4-8	1-5	0
	12-15	12-13	8-11	6-9	4-7	1-5	0

How to Quit:
A Step-by-Step Guide

When you're ready to quit smoking for good, here are some step-by-step suggestions designed to help you succeed. They're gleaned from thousands of people who have made that difficult U-turn on tobacco road.

STEP 1: ARE YOU READY?

You've taken the Stages of Change Test on page 6, and you're sure you're ready and willing to quit. If you scored 70 percent or higher on the Quit-Smoking Confidence Questionnaire, page 182, it's likely that you can quit on your own. If you scored lower, seek out a smoking-cessation program that offers plenty of support.

STEP 2: WHAT HELP DO YOU NEED?

If you normally smoke more than 25 cigarettes a day, find it difficult to go without smoking for longer than an hour, and smoke as soon as you get up in the morning, you'd likely benefit from the nicotine chewing gum or patch. If you need help, get it well in advance of your quit date.

STEP 3: GET MORAL SUPPORT

Before you quit, it's vital to get full support from your family, coworkers, friends, and doctor. Those closest to you can make it easier—or more difficult—to quit smoking, so be sure to gather support where you can find it. Try to ignore those who attempt to sabotage you or don't support you.

STEP 4: PROMISE YOURSELF

Make a formal commitment to quit smoking. Sign a contract with a friend, quitting buddy, or health-care professional, outlining your determination to quit on a certain date. This will help you focus and boost your chances of success.

STEP 5: REVIEW YOUR GAME PLAN

Identify high-risk situations and practice techniques to get you through them. Gather all your quit-smoking tools: exercise clothes, snacks and chewables, activities to keep you busy, and phone numbers of friends to call.

STEP 6: CHOOSE A METHOD

There are two ways to quit smoking: cold turkey, which is quitting all at once, or the gradual-reduction plan, which is smoking fewer cigarettes every day until you've quit. Statistics show that, by far, the cold-turkey method is the most successful.

QUITTING COLD TURKEY

To quit cold turkey, you set a definite quit date within the next week—a date on which you will suddenly stop smoking for good. During the days before this quit date, keep track of the number of cigarettes you smoke, using the following method: Wrap your cigarette packs in plain paper fastened with a rubber band. Each time you want a cigarette, unwrap the paper and write two facts on it: the time and what you are doing. For example:

CIGARETTE	TIME	WHAT YOU ARE DOING
#1	7:30 A.M.	Having coffee
#2	8:05 A.M.	Driving to work
#3	9:45 A.M.	Coffee break at work

Keeping this record helps you in several ways: It keeps you from automatically reaching for a cigarette, it makes smoking slightly more difficult, and it helps you become aware of the situations and people that may trigger you to smoke. When you do quit, you will know about these situations in advance and be able to take measures to help you handle them without smoking.

QUITTING GRADUALLY

If you decide to cut down gradually, certain techniques are better than others. It's more effective to reduce your nicotine intake by at least half each time you cut down. Do it quickly, finishing in no more than seven days.

Here are several strategies that can be effective:

- *Quit in four parts.* The first day, reduce the number of cigarettes you smoke by half. In two more days, cut it down again by half. Cut in half again two days after that. On your quit day, stop altogether. For example, if you smoke 30 cigarettes a day, cut that to 15 on the first day, 7 or 8 two days later, and 2 or 3 two days after that. Stop smoking on the seventh day.

- *Switch brands.* Immediately switch to a brand containing 50 percent or less nicotine than your present brand, and smoke the new brand for two days. Then find a brand that has half the nicotine of that brand, and use that for two days. Two days later, cut down on the number of cigarettes you smoke by half. On the seventh day, quit entirely.

- *Percentage slashing.* On the first day, reduce the percentage of each cigarette you smoke by half. In two days, smoke no more than a quarter of each cigarette. Two days after that, cut down the number of cigarettes you smoke by half and smoke no more than a quarter of those. Be aware that this method clearly takes more self-discipline than the other two.

If you can't quit by using these techniques, you might as well quit cold turkey. Or consider using nicotine gum or the patch or joining a formal smoking-cessation program.

STEP 7: FOLLOW A DAILY PROGRAM

This daily program will help you change your behavior and quit smoking. Follow it for *at least six weeks*. You can change it around to fit with your schedule, but remember that it's vital to walk or exercise three times a day, eat regularly, and have a pleasure replacement (doing something pleasurable to replace the pleasure of cigarettes) at least once a day.

DAILY PROGRAM	
TIME	ACTION
Morning	Breakfast
Midmorning	5-minute walk or exericse
Lunchtime	15-minute walk or exercise Lunch
Midafternoon	Snack (if hungry) 15-minute walk or exercise
Dinnertime	Dinner
After dinner	Pleasure replacement

STEP 8: REVIEW THE MAJOR COPING STRATEGIES

They're tried and true. The following strategies can help get you through the toughest part of quitting. All of them are important. *Don't ignore even one.*

PHYSICAL ACTIVITY

Regular physical activity gives you something to concentrate on besides nicotine urges. It gives you something to do. It gives you energy, burns calories, and helps you concentrate, relax, and feel less stressed and irritable.

Walking is the easiest form of physical activity because it works with any schedule. Moderate exercise, such as walking, is safe for almost everyone. In general, if you are too breathless to hold a conversation while you exercise, slow down. Read the chapter on physical activity, page 115. It's filled with great ideas on how to get the most out of exercise. This chapter not only will help you quit smoking but also can lead to a lifetime love affair with physical activity.

EATING

Food can have a powerful effect in fighting the urge to smoke. Eating regular meals will help you maintain your body's energy stores so you feel less tired. It also helps you tolerate stress and curbs that "empty" feeling. Furthermore, new taste sensations will help make up for losing the pleasure of smoking.

Initially you may gain a little weight because your metabolism slows down when you're off nicotine. The average smoker, however, gains only six pounds—no big deal when compared to the gargantuan health risk of smoking. If it's a choice between a cigarette and a candy bar, *pick the candy bar.* You can lose weight later.

Here's a stop-smoking eating plan that works:

- *Don't diet or count calories.* Eat full, nutritious meals and snacks during the quitting process. Even splurge a little. Better too much food than too little at this critical time.

- *Don't even think about skipping meals.* This is especially true of breakfast. If you're hungry, you're risking a relapse. Don't go there.

- *Exercise regularly.* It will help take care of excess calories.

- *Stock up on ex-smoker foods.* Those are foods that give you something to do with your mouth (gum, crackers, apples, popcorn), something to do with your hands (nuts in the shell, oranges, sunflower seeds, grapes with seeds), and something to help you fight smoking urges (sweet foods). Choose sweet foods that are low in fat—angel food cake, fresh and dried fruits, hard candies, jelly beans, and sorbets. They'll give you the sweet taste ex-smokers crave with much fewer calories than high-fat sweets, such as most cakes, cookies, and ice creams.

Remember: *Quitting smoking is your first priority.* You can lose weight later.

ALTERNATIVE PLEASURES

We discussed this earlier, but alternative pleasures can't be overemphasized. When you quit smoking, you feel intense *deprivation.* Something must replace that. Seek clear, vivid alternative pleasures to replace this deprived feeling. You must treat yourself to at least one alternative pleasure every day.

It can be anything that makes you feel decadent. Treat yourself to a massage, read part of a book, attend a concert or sports event, spend time outdoors, buy new clothes, cook your favorite foods, try a new restaurant, watch television or rent a fun video, buy a new CD—the list is endless. Make pampering yourself at least once every day part of your plan. *This is not optional.* It is critical to your success.

RELAPSE STRATEGIES

Many situations, events, and feelings—including drinking a cup of coffee, seeing someone else smoke, feeling stress, having an alcoholic drink, even the "high" of feeling good—can trigger your desire to smoke. Review the situational strategies outlined on page 183 and be ready with your relapse-prevention strategies. *A good offense is the best defense.*

STRESS MANAGEMENT

Smokers who relapse often report that the culprit was a stressful situation. That's why it's important to do everything you can to reduce the stress and tension in your life during the first few months after quitting.

Besides walking or other exercise, relaxation helps immeasurably. For example, meditation has been known to lower heart rate and blood pressure, put you in a restful frame of mind, and relax your muscles. Those are exactly the responses you want. You can meditate, do biofeedback, listen to music, try self-hypnosis, or do any number of other techniques to get this deep relaxation. Set aside 15 to 20 minutes a day for the next six weeks.

Experts say that laughter also works to reduce tension. Pull out those comedy videos, watch funny sit-coms, or read humorous books. You could also take up a soothing hobby, such as needlework, model making, or other crafts. Choose something you can turn to instantly when the urge to smoke is strong.

Take a vacation from worry. Try to put aside whatever is worrying you. It'll keep until you've quit smoking. Better yet, take an actual vacation. Lots of smokers have quit simply by leaving town—and everyday stress—behind. If these efforts fail, try a formal stress-management program. Whatever it takes, keep your stress to a minimum. Low stress means greater success.

HOW TO TURN A RELAPSE AROUND

Relapses are almost inevitable. Here's how to handle them successfully:

- Treat the relapse as temporary. It's just part of the process.

- Stop smoking immediately.

- Throw away all cigarettes, ashtrays, and lighters.

- Get a piece of paper and write down three reasons for quitting and three reasons for starting to smoke again. Look at your list and make your decision. Then proceed accordingly. Whatever you decide, at least you'll do it *consciously*.

HOW TO QUIT SMOKING:
AN AT-A-GLANCE CHECKLIST

___Make sure you're ready to quit.

___Set a quit date within the next week.

___Prepare your support system (family, friends, tools, classes, gum, etc.).

___Sign your quit-smoking contract in the presence of a supportive family member, friend, or health-care professional.

___During the days before you quit, keep track of the number of cigarettes you smoke each day and the circumstances in which you smoke them.

___The evening before your quit day, get rid of all your cigarettes, lighters, and ashtrays.

___On your quit day, keep to a program of regular meals and healthful snacks, exercise, stress reduction, and fun activities.

___Plan alternative pleasures at least daily. These intensely pleasurable activities help you overcome the feeling of deprivation when you no longer have cigarettes for comfort.

___Keep busy; change your surroundings; deeply relax; talk to friends.

___Memorize and continually review your situational strategies to prevent relapse.

__If you do relapse, stop smoking again
immediately and throw away all cigarettes.
Write down three reasons for quitting and
three reasons for starting again. Then make
your decision.

NO-SMOKING CONTRACT

Before you start the quitting process, sign this contract in front of a witness. The witness can be a
spouse, relative, close friend, or health-care professional—somebody who will stand by you if you
need help.

I, _____ , promise that I will re-
main a nonsmoker for the next year.

If by any chance I should slip up, I will immediately
contact the witness whose name appears below.
With his or her help, I will return to my life as a
nonsmoker.

Signed _____   Date _____

Witness _____   Date _____

If you do have a slip, think of it as that: a slip. It
doesn't mean you're a failure, and it doesn't mean
you're a smoker again. See "How to Turn a Relapse
Around," page 218. Then get right back on track as a
nonsmoker.

healthy,
WEALTHY,
AND WISE
how to work with your doctor to stay well

"EVEN IF YOU'RE ON
THE RIGHT TRACK, YOU'LL GET RUN
OVER IF YOU JUST SIT THERE."
— MARK TWAIN

Who's in **Charge** Here?

We'll give you a hint: It's not your doctor, even though your doctor is your chief consultant. The truth is, you're in charge. It's up to you to be a champion for your own health care. Besides using this book to help you quit smoking, eat more healthfully, and get more exercise, we want you to remember that you're in control of your own well-being at home and at the doctor's office.

Your first area of responsibility? Get regular checkups. It's only smart to keep tabs on your blood pressure, blood cholesterol, and blood sugar levels. Because high blood pressure, elevated cholesterol levels, and diabetes usually have no symptoms until damage is done, you'll want to monitor these indicators on a regular basis. Make sure you know how your general health checks out and what conditions need watching or treatment.

WHAT KIND OF TESTS DO YOU NEED?

AGE	HOW OFTEN
GENERAL PHYSICAL EXAM	
20 to 60	Every 5 years
61 to 75	Every 2 years
After 75	Every year
BLOOD PRESSURE	
20 and older	Every 2 years
• If apparently healthy or less than 130 over less than 85 mm Hg	
• If high risk or 130 to139 over 85 to 89 mm Hg	Every year
• If 140 to 159 over 90 to 99 mm Hg	Confirm within 2 months and monitor
TOTAL CHOLESTEROL	
2 and older	At age 2 and then every year
• If family history of heart disease, stroke, or high cholesterol	
TOTAL CHOLESTEROL AND HDL	
20 through 60	Every 5 years
• If apparently healthy	
20 and older	Every year
• If high risk: total cholesterol 200 to 239 mg/dl and HDL less than 35 mg/dl or with 2 or more other risk factors or with cholesterol 240 mg/dl or higher	

AGE	HOW OFTEN
61 and older • If apparently healthy	Every 5 years
FASTING BLOOD SUGAR 20 to 75	Every 5 years
ELECTROCARDIOGRAM (ECG) Adult • If high risk: 2 OR more risk factors and family history of early heart disease	One by age 40 for a baseline
EXERCISE TEST Adult • If high risk: 2 or more risk factors or presence of diabetes or family history of early heart disease or those over 40 who plan a vigorous exercise program or those who would endanger public safety if they experienced sudden cardiac events	Frequency should be determined by your doctor based on goals for prevention, treatment, or monitoring

You need to take charge of your health yourself because those decisions are too important to leave to anyone else. Here are some ways you can work with your health-care provider:

• Explain that you want to help make the decisions about your health.

• Gather information to understand what your doctor is saying and recommending.

- Before agreeing to a medication, test, or lifestyle change, ask your doctor why he or she is recommending it and how it will help you.

- Ask about treatment options and state which you prefer.

- Tell your health-care provider exactly what you expect from a treatment and ask whether your expectations are realistic.

- Bring along lists of your current medications, including over-the-counter medicines, vitamins, and dietary supplements.

---

bergen's story:
AN OUNCE OF PREVENTION

"My wife, Jane, and I are from the old school," said Bergen, a retired schoolteacher. "We did whatever the doctor said and didn't ask questions. It was one-way communication only. It was like that for years, until Jane had a bad drug reaction. Boy, did we change our tune."

From that day on, Bergen and Jane took personal responsibility for their health. Not only do they question their health-care provider about diagnosis and treatment, but they also ask their pharmacist about their medications. In addition, they look up medicines on the Internet and study at the library.

"We don't take *aspirin* without knowing why," said Bergen. "I can tell you every possible side effect of my blood-pressure medicine. I know what to look for, whether it's working, even how it works. Jane and I will never fly blind again."

Information Highway

Take advantage of all the sources of information you have at hand, including the library and local health organizations. You base your health-care choices on what you know—so it's up to you to make the most of taking charge. Your doctor can help you, but ultimately it's your decision how to manage your own health.

If you have access to the Internet, use the Web to research any health problem you may have and the medicines used to treat it. You'll be in good company. One poll reports that 60 million adults used the Internet to find health information in 1998.

donna's story:
COMPUTER SUPPORT

"When I was first diagnosed with diabetes, I totally panicked," said Donna, who worked in the purchasing department of a large oil company. "I thought I'd lose a foot or go blind. Even though my doctor said that we'd caught it early and it was treatable, I was really scared."

Donna decided to research the disease online. She was amazed at the possibilities. The more Donna read about the disease, the more hope she had for her own treatment.

"I got with the program," she said. "I changed my lifestyle and my eating habits and began my new walking plan. And I've been meticulous about taking medication. It was a long haul, but the newsgroups and chat groups dealing with this illness were wonderfully supportive. I've had my diabetes under control for two years. The support I received on the Internet was vital to my peace of mind."

When it comes to taking charge of your health, all you need is enough support to give you that little extra measure of courage. You can get this kind of support from individuals and groups both in person and on the Internet. In cyberspace, you can also find a world of information geared to help you stop smoking, lose weight, get more exercise, and manage prescription medicines.

Be choosy about information you see on the Internet. Anyone can post notices, so misinformation is plentiful. Just as you would do in reading printed material, choose to believe reliable authorities. These sites will give you the tips, tools, and programs you need to succeed. In fact, feel free to start with the medication section of our website at www.american-heart.org/CAP.

If you're a heart patient, you can get support from Mended Hearts, Inc., a national network of recovered heart patients. Visit the website at www.mendedhearts.org, or to find a Mended Hearts chapter in your area, call the American Heart Association at 1-800-AHA-USA1 (1-800-242-8721).

Stroke survivors can find information from the American Stroke Association at www.strokeassociation.org or by calling 1-888-4-STROKE; ask for the Stroke Family Support Network. Stroke survivors and caregivers on the network offer information and referrals, including contact information for a stroke support group near you.

Similar sources of information on the Internet and similar support groups are available for other diseases. Seek these out—it's all part of taking charge.

Just What the Doctor Ordered

Now that you know where you stand, it's time to become an active partner in your health care. As we've said, don't be shy—when a doctor prescribes a medication for you, ask about the diagnosis and choice of treatment. Make sure you understand what the medicine will do. Take the following questions, plus pen and paper, to every doctor's appointment.

MEDICATION Q & A

1. What is the name of the medication, and what is it supposed to do?

2. How and when do I take it and for how long? What if I miss a dose?

3. What foods, drinks, or other medications or activities should I avoid when taking this medicine? (Be sure to cite any allergic reactions you've had from any medicine.)

4. Will this prescription work safely with my current prescription and nonprescription medications? (Always carry a list of all current medications in your billfold, or carry all the bottles with you in a bag when you visit the doctor.)

5. What possible side effects could I experience, and what should I do if I experience them?

6. Is there any written information available on this medicine?

Most doctors welcome your active interest and participation in the diagnosis and treatment process. Don't think that you are questioning the doctor's authority —you're getting information you need.

TAKE AS DIRECTED

If you're one of the millions of Americans taking prescription drugs, you need to know why taking your medications every day is more than a good idea—it's vitally important to your treatment.

If you have follow-up or unanswered questions after discussing your medication with your doctor, be sure to ask your pharmacist. You may wonder whether the medicine should be taken with a meal or on an empty stomach. If you take it once a day, is it better to take it in the morning or at bedtime? Most pharmacies have a consultation or counseling area where you can meet with the pharmacist to get information that is specific for you.

About 20 percent of all prescriptions are never filled. Theoretically, at least, this means 20 percent of all people with diagnosed chronic conditions such as high blood pressure, diabetes, and high blood cholesterol are not getting their prescribed treatment.

Unfortunately, ignoring these conditions will not make them go away. Instead, this puts these untreated people in danger.

RX FACT

The top two classes of medicines prescribed in 1998 were those that treat high blood pressure and depression.

Even when people conscientiously get their prescriptions filled, too often they stop taking their drugs abruptly if they begin to feel bad—or if they start feeling better. In fact, studies show that almost half of all prescription drugs are *not taken as prescribed* and thus are much less effective than they might have been.

For example, high-blood-pressure drugs often make you feel bad at first. That's no reason to abruptly stop taking them. If you do, your blood pressure will once again be uncontrolled, placing you at risk for stroke, kidney failure, or heart attack. Instead of stopping the medication, talk with your doctor and find a drug that will work without the side effects.

Another common problem is failure to take antibiotics for the entire time period prescribed. Even though you usually start feeling better in a few days, it takes a week or more to kill off most bacteria. When you stop the medicine as soon as you begin to feel better, you've killed only some of the bacteria. The remaining bacteria can start freely reproducing again, and the condition may return. Or, worse, the bacteria could develop resistance to the medicine, so the drug may not work next time.

Simply *forgetting a dose* is another obvious reason why people don't follow through with their prescriptions as directed.

- To help you remember to take bedtime medicines, keep them near your toothpaste or travel alarm—somewhere you'll definitely go before retiring. Try to pair medicines with some other activity you'll be doing without fail—put them near the breakfast dishes for morning medicines or with the salt and pepper shakers if the medicines will be taken with meals.

- Try posting sticky notes on your bathroom mirror to remind you of a morning pill. Sticky notes work best for one-time-only reminders.

- Use pill boxes or other organizers to keep track if you need several medications each day (see the section on organizers in "Pill-Taking 101," page 234).

HEADS UP, BABY BOOMERS!

If you thought that only *older* Americans forget their medications, you're wrong. Researchers have found that older Americans make the *fewest* errors. Middle-age adults make the most. It seems that busy lifestyles and middle age are the greatest determinants of risk.

PILL-TAKING 101

Being in charge means finding a way to take your medicines that works with your lifestyle. Feel free to talk about the following concerns with your health-care provider.

COSTS

If you're on a limited budget, let your doctor or health-care provider know that cost is an issue. A less costly medicine may be available. If you can't afford a drug you need, ask your health-care provider about manufacturer's aid. Most major drug companies have programs that give medications to patients who don't have insurance or can't pay for medicine. In these cases, the doctor must apply for you.

CONVENIENCE

If doctor and pharmacy visits are difficult to schedule or to reach, talk to your health-care professional. You may be able to schedule visits at a time that works better for you and have your medications delivered by the pharmacy or by mail.

ORGANIZERS

Are you taking several medications throughout the day? If so, you may want to get organized. Consider writing your medication times on a daily calendar.

After you take the medicine, place a check mark next to its name on the calendar.

You can also buy an inexpensive plastic pill box with a compartment for each day of the week. Put a week's worth of all your daily pills in the pill box. Some even have three or four pill slots per day, one each for morning, afternoon, evening, and bedtime. If you take pills at only two different times, have two boxes, one for morning and one for evening. Pill boxes really take the guesswork out of "Did I take my medicine today?"

This may sound low-tech, but it works: Ask a family member or buddy to remind you to take your medication. Are high-tech solutions more your thing? Try a computerized pill box. It will alert you when it's time to take a pill and when you need to get a refill.

Fortunately, dozens of creative tools are available to help you remember your medicine. Here are just a few of them:

- E-mail and beeper services
- Wristwatches with alarms
- Drug-reminder charts
- Pill calendars
- Special medication dispensers (ask your pharmacist)
- Compartmentalized pill boxes

- Unit dose packages (ask your pharmacist)
- Stickers
- Diaries
- Subscription computer health programs

DRUG REACTIONS

Not only is it important to take your medicine as prescribed, it's also wise to ask your doctor how to avoid drug reactions. Also, when you get a new prescription, check with your pharmacist to see if it will interact with any of the drugs you're already taking. In 1994, researchers found that more than two million hospitalized patients had serious adverse drug reactions. When you consider that more than 3 billion retail prescriptions were filled in 1999, you can see how easy it would be to become a statistic.

---

glenda's story:
A PAINFUL LESSON

"I sprained my ankle real bad on a Saturday," said Glenda, "and by Sunday, it was really throbbing. My husband had some old pain medication, so I thought, 'Maybe this will help.' That was a big mistake. Turns out I was allergic to it. Got the worst case of hives you ever saw. I was in the emergency room for three hours."

Actually, Glenda was lucky. The resident who treated her told her about a man who had such a severe allergy to a prescription drug that his lips swelled up to twice their normal size, his trachea closed, and he couldn't breathe. He was rushed to the hospital by ambulance and barely made it in time.

"I tell you what," said Glenda, "I learned my lesson. I'm not taking anything—*not anything*—unless I know it's safe for me."

MEDICATION-MISTAKE BUSTERS

You've no doubt read the horror stories of people accidentally taking the wrong medication or mixing medications and creating adverse effects. Here are some tips that will help you steer clear of these medicine-related mix-ups.

- Make a list of medications you're taking. Include the dose, how often you take it, the imprint on the capsule, and the name of the pharmacy that filled the prescription. Keep your medication list updated.

- List any over-the-counter medications, vitamins, nutritional supplements, or herbal products you take regularly.

- List your medication and food allergies.

- Keep medicines in their original containers. Many pills look alike; when you keep them in their original containers, you'll know which is which and how to take them.

- Never take someone else's medication. You don't know how it will interact with your medication, the dosage may be wrong for you, or you may be allergic to it.

- Read the label every time you take a drug to make sure you're taking the right dose and following the instructions.

- Turn on the lights every time you take a drug. You don't want to accidentally take the wrong thing in the middle of the night.

- Allow plenty of time for refills, so you won't run out.

- Don't store your medicines in the bathroom or in direct sunlight. Humidity, light, and heat can affect drug potency. Store your medicines as the bottle directs. For example, nitroglycerin comes in a dark bottle because it is so sensitive to light. It must be kept in a dark, airtight bottle in a cabinet.

- Keep medication for people separate from medication for pets. Amazingly, mix-ups are common and can be dangerous.

- Don't keep tubes of ointments near your toothpaste. Don't keep glue bottles near your eye or ear drops. They look and feel alike when you grab quickly.

- Flush any old medication down the toilet. Certain drugs become toxic after their expiration date. Children and pets can retrieve medications thrown in a wastebasket.

- Don't chew, crush, or break any medication unless instructed to do so. Otherwise, the drug may be absorbed too quickly, which may make you sick or prevent it from working correctly.

- Always use the correct dosage cup for liquid medication. Don't mix and match them.

- Always take your medicines exactly as prescribed. That's how they're most effective.

MEDICATION RULES OF THE ROAD

As part of taking responsibility for your health, be aware of the basic rules of how to take medications safely and get the most benefit.

- Don't drink alcohol with any prescription drug until you check with your doctor or pharmacist.

- If you're pregnant or breast-feeding, make sure the medicine will not affect the health of the baby.

- Tell your doctor before stopping or starting any medication.

- When you ask your doctor or pharmacist about your medications, take notes! It's impossible to remember everything.

- Carefully read the description that comes with the medication, including side effects and warnings. Call your pharmacist or doctor to double-check if you have questions about any aspect of the medicine or dosage. (Only 12 percent of Americans read this literature. If you're one of them, you're more likely to avoid being an adverse-drug-reaction statistic.)

- If you must stop taking your medication for any reason, tell your health-care provider. He or she may base future decisions about your health care on your experience with this medicine.

---

wally's story:
PERSONALIZED REMINDER

A retired travel agent and heart patient, Wally took a whole variety of medicines— each at a different time of the day. He took medications for gout, high blood cholesterol, irregular heart rhythm, and digestion; he also took a blood thinner and a diuretic. He asked a lot of questions until he was sure he understood what each one did and how they worked together, but he had one problem that made him feel out of control.

"I could remember which ones I needed in the morning and at night," said Wally. "But I couldn't for the life of me remember my four o'clock heart pill. I tried leaving notes for myself and programming my brain to alert me. Nothing worked."

One day Wally found the perfect pill-taking reminder in a catalog: a pocket-size alarm that you could program with the date and time you wanted a reminder. Then you could record, in your own voice, exactly the message you wanted to hear.

"I programmed the device to beep at four o'clock every day," said Wally. "I recorded my own voice saying, 'Take your heart pill.' Sure enough, every afternoon at four, no matter where I was, the alarm sounded and I heard my own voice reminding me to take the pill. It was perfect." Today, Wally carries that alarm in his pocket wherever he goes—along with the pills he needs.

The voice reminder works perfectly for Wally, and the same idea can work for you too. No matter what your personal situation, you can be in control. Like Wally, all you have to do is *listen to your own voice* to take charge of your health!

you can
TAKE IT
FROM HERE!
we're behind you all the way

"SUCCESS IS A LITTLE LIKE
WRESTLING A GORILLA. YOU DON'T
QUIT WHEN YOU'RE TIRED—YOU
QUIT WHEN THE GORILLA IS TIRED."

—ROBERT STRAUSS

CHANGING YOUR LIFE FOR THE BETTER IS ONE OF THE GREAT PRIZES OF LIFE. On these pages, we hope you have seen that making a fresh start *can* be done. People can—and do—quit smoking, lose weight, and become more physically active every day. And they do it permanently. They anchor the changes so firmly to their lives that the new lifestyle becomes a part of who they actually are. They have become healthy, slender, nonsmoking, physically active people. That's just how it is.

Ask anybody who's done it. Although they may use different words, you'll hear that they have five things in common.

Five Steps to **Success**

1. *Just say yes.* You can do it! The event that enables you to do it is the decision in your brain that you're going to do it. This decision gives you the power to do it. You'll know when you've decided. It's the difference between "I kind of want to" and "I'm going to."

2. *Set realistic goals.* Changing your life is not torture. It's a choice to make the changes you want one step at a time. Realize that it takes time to change habits. Close the door on the past and open it to your new future.

3. *It's okay to mess up.* Nobody's perfect. Instead of concentrating on your flaws, hone in on your assets, talents, and abilities. Mistakes are part of life. No one is exempt, not even you. Just get back on your plan and go on.

4. *Nip it in the bud.* You'll be tempted to return to your old life. It's going to happen. If you're to succeed, you'll have to set your own internal alarm, an automatic shutoff that returns you to your new path. For some, the warning light is gaining an extra three pounds. The reaction? To immediately start working to lose the extra weight. For others, it's smelling cigarette smoke in a crowded bar, so they leave immediately. For still others, it's a long weekend without exercise, so on Monday, they lace up their walking shoes and hit the track. People who have changed their lifestyle know not to let temptation or a slipup change their habits. They always, *always* stop and recommit to their new life.

5. *Face your pain*. Too many people live unsatisfying lives because they won't look at their own pain, their own "shadow side." Fear—even fear of facing your own feelings—can keep you from getting the life you want. Learn to feel, and deal with, the pain and negativity in your life. Get help if you need it. Unless you face your shadow side, you won't live your own life. It will live you.

Hang On to This Book

Changing your life is done in stages. You may want to quit smoking today; then next January find you want to get more exercise. The point is, keep this book handy on your bookshelf. Return to it for support and a refresher. When the going gets rough, review the strategies. If you haven't read the weight-loss chapter because your main interest is quitting smoking, no problem. Perhaps you'll find you want to lose 15 pounds next year. Turn to that chapter for help and encouragement when you're ready.

Holly, an executive secretary in a bank, lost 34 pounds at age 40 and has kept it off for seven years. Recently, she reminisced about how her decision to make a fresh start continues to reap rich rewards. "I feel better and look better," said Holly. "People think I'm about forty. That's flattering, but it's not what I like most. The thing I love about finally having more energy and being slender is that I call the shots. Nothing owns me but me. That's my definition of success."

We wish you that kind of success and more. You can do it!

FOR FURTHER INFORMATION

For further information about American Heart Association programs and services, call 1-800-AHA-USA1 (1-800-242-8721) or contact us online at www.americanheart.org. For information about the American Stroke Association, a division of the American Heart Association, call 1-888-4STROKE (1-888-478-7653).

NATIONAL CENTER

American Heart Association
7272 Greenville Avenue
Dallas, TX 75231-4596
214-373-6300

OPERATING UNITS OF THE NATIONAL CENTER

Office of Public Advocacy
Washington, DC

American Heart Association, Hawaii
Honolulu, HI

AFFILIATES

Desert/Mountain Affiliate
Arizona, Colorado, New Mexico, Wyoming
Denver, CO

Florida/Puerto Rico Affiliate
St. Petersburg, FL

Heartland Affiliate
Arkansas, Iowa, Kansas, Missouri, Nebraska,
    Oklahoma
Topeka, KS

Heritage Affiliate
Connecticut, Long Island, New Jersey, New
    York City
New York, NY

Mid-Atlantic Affiliate
District of Columbia, Maryland, North
    Carolina, South Carolina, Virginia
Glen Allen, VA

Midwest Affiliate
Illinois, Indiana, Michigan
Chicago, IL

New England Affiliate
Maine, Massachusetts, New Hampshire,
    Rhode Island, Vermont
Framingham, MA

New York State Affiliate
Syracuse, NY

Northland Affiliate
Minnesota, North Dakota, South Dakota,
   Wisconsin
Minneapolis, MN

Northwest Affiliate
Alaska, Idaho, Montana, Oregon, Washington
Seattle, WA

Ohio Valley Affiliate
Kentucky, Ohio, West Virginia
Columbus, OH

Pennsylvania/Delaware Affiliate
Delaware, Pennsylvania
Wormleysburg, PA

Southeast Affiliate
Alabama, Georgia, Louisiana, Mississippi,
   Tennessee
Marietta, GA

Texas Affiliate
Austin, TX

Western States Affiliate
California, Nevada, Utah
Los Angeles, CA

INDEX